Evaluation
in
Physical Education

Evaluation in Physical Education

Mary Jane Haskins

Associate Professor of Physical Education
Lamar State College of Technology
Beaumont, Texas

WM. C. BROWN COMPANY PUBLISHERS
Dubuque, Iowa

CONSULTING EDITORS

PHYSICAL EDUCATION

Aileene Lockhart
University of Southern California

PARKS AND RECREATION

David Gray
California State College, Long Beach

HEALTH

Robert Kaplan
Ohio State University

Contents

Page

Preface vii

Chapter

1 Introduction.................................. 1
   Objectives and Purpose of
   Measurement and Evaluation 1

2 Tests in Physical Education 6
   Test Selection 6
   Strength 9
   Endurance 13
   Physical Fitness 14
   Motor Ability 33
   Posture 45
   The Concomitants 52
      Social Adjustment 52
      Behavior 54
      Attitude 59
      Sportsmanship 63
   Sports Skill Testing 78
      Archery 78
      Badminton 85
      Basketball 91
      Field Hockey 109
      Football 115
      Golf 132
      Soccer 137
      Softball 141
      Swimming 160
      Tennis 165

v

Chapter   Page

      Volleyball 168
      Game Performance Testing 177

3   Rating Scales and Check Lists 180
      Skills Inventory 186
      Construction of Rating Scales and Check Lists 186
      Hints on Administration of Rating Scales 190

4   Administrative Procedures in the Testing Program 192
      Test Selection 192
      Space and Time Planning 193
      Preparation of Score Cards 196
      Assistants 197
      Instructions 198
      Scoring 198
      Preparation of Test Area and Equipment 198
      Orient the Students 199
      After Testing 199

5   Statistical Procedures 200
      Measures of Central Tendency 201
         The Mean 201
         The Median 203
         The Mode 203
      The Normal Curve 204
      The Standard Deviation—A Measure of Variability 205
      Calculation of the Standard Deviation 206
      Standard Scores and Percentiles 211
         Sigma, Hull, and T-Scales 212
         Percentiles 214
      Reliability of the Mean 216
         The Standard Error of the Mean (SE_m) 218
      Significance of the Difference Between Means 219
         The Standard Error of the
         Difference Between Means (SE_D) 219
         The Critical Ratio (t) 222
      Correlation 224
      Standard Error of the Difference
      Between Correlated Means 230
      Standard Error of the Difference
      Between Differences 233
      The Experimental Design 234
         Clues in Experimental Design 236

Chapter   Page

  6 Test Construction 239
   Skill Test Construction 239
   Construction of Written Tests 241
   Construction of Written Test Questions 241
    Alternate Response 241
    Matching 243
    Short Answer and Completion 247
    Multiple Choice 248
    Special Formats: Diagram, Drawings, Etc. 249
    Essay 250
   Test Construction 250
   Test Analysis 253
   Scoring and Answer Sheets 259

  7 Grading 262
   Measurable Factors 263
   Subjective Evaluation 265
   Methods of Assigning Grades 267
    The Twelve Point Grading Scale 269
    Grading Systems 270

  8 Conclusion 273
   Philosophy and Evaluation 275

  Bibliography 277

  Appendix 287

Preface

"Is my program and are my methods providing the physical education experiences which will meet the needs of my students?" Physical education has the potential to meet many student needs in the area of biological, neuro-muscular, personal-social, and interpretative development. It is difficult to secure objective evidence of growth in some of these areas. Many facets of physical education do not lend themselves easily to objective measurement: Therefore the instructor of physical education should understand and possess skills in both objective and subjective evaluation. It is not the purpose of this text to influence the prospective teacher toward providing a program which is easily measured, but rather to provide him with the skills and tools which will make it possible for him to evaluate a broadly conceived program in a manner which will be defensible and which will provide evidence of its effectiveness.

Most professional students in physical education do not enter the curriculum with an extensive background in mathematics. Since the traditional approach to measurement, particularly the statistical handling and interpretation of results, fails to encourage these students, the problem-solving approach is utilized here and emphasis is given to development of a philosophy of evaluation.

The text is written in a logical sequence with frequent examples and sample problems. A great deal of factual information (easily available in other sources) has been purposefully omitted to allow for the problem-solving approach; however sufficient materials are included so that another source is not necessary to a course in Measurement and Evaluation.

It is hoped that this approach will appeal to the professional student and that its use will ease his difficulties with the subject. Evaluation is a basic tool which all teachers must use in arriving at the appraisals, interpretations and judgments which they daily make. It is hoped that these evaluations will be made as thoughtfully and objectively as possible.

chapter

1

Introduction

Measurement as the term is used here entails assigning a quantitative symbol or score to a student's capability in a quality being measured. *Evaluation* gives value to that score, assessing its meaning and importance within the total structure of our objectives. Measurement is relatively simple, merely requiring careful adherence to set specifications and proper use of a tool, while evaluation demands philosophy, well thought out objectives, and understanding of the values and limitations of tools of measurement.

Objectives and Purposes of Measurement and Evaluation

One essential to effective teaching is that the teacher and the students understand the objectives of the course. It therefore seems appropriate to begin this book with a list of the objectives which it is hoped the student will achieve from its study.

1. Understand the function of testing and measurement.
2. Be able to evaluate results.
3. Be able to recognize and write good questions.
4. Be able to administer tests and explain their results.
5. Recognize the values and limitations of tests, and the interpretation of results.
6. Be able to use elementary statistical procedures and understand their limitations and uses.
7. Become familiar with tests and testing procedures in physical education.
8. Develop a philosophy about evaluation.
9. Develop an experimental outlook.
10. Be able to devise an experimental design, follow it through, and interpret the results.

Determining what the student's objectives may be is not the function of this text. The student will certainly be exposed to varying philosophies of physical education and eventually will develop his own personal reference point. His philosophy will determine his objectives and, particularly, the amount of emphasis he will place on his various objectives. We measure and evaluate according to our objectives. For the sake of organization the general objectives for physical education adopted by the AAHPER are used here to classify the various types of measurement available to the teacher of physical education. These objectives and the qualities to be measured are

1. Organic development involving strength, power, physical fitness, cardiovascular endurance.
2. Neuro-muscular development involving coordination, motor ability, sport and movement skills.
3. Personal-social development involving attitude, sportsmanship, leadership, social grace, ideals, democratic behavior.
4. Interpretive development involving knowledges, strategies, understandings.

Perhaps the main purpose of evaluation should be to improve learning, and to do this it is necessary to find out about our students, our methods, and our programs. Is our program and are our methods successful in promoting student growth in the areas encompassed by our objectives? In order to answer this question we must evaluate and to do that we need to measure. There are several purposes to measurement: one is to classify students in order to group them in such a way as to provide optimum learning conditions; a second is to determine the status of our students so that our program can be constructed to best meet their needs; a third purpose is to evaluate the instructor's methods; a fourth is to provide motivation for teacher and student improvement; and fifth, to provide a basis for grading, for if grades are to be given in physical education then we must be able to explain and justify those grades.

Let us take an example: suppose that we believe physical education is well suited to the development of physical fitness, and that we also believe this objective can be reached through the development of sports skills. We believe that these will provide pleasure and personal satisfactions to the extent that the student will continue to participate in those skills and therefore they will continue to contribute to his physical fitness. (You may care to refer to studies which indicate that practice of sports skills does develop and maintain physical fitness).[4] Since physical fitness is one of our objectives we select a valid and reliable test, administer it to our students early in the program and at the end of the course of study. We now have two sets of fitness scores—what do they mean? How did student A compare with the others in the class? With national norms? Was he below average on the broad jump for example? Could that have affected his ability to rebound in basketball? Was he still below average at the end of the course, or had he improved his standing? Did this inability cause him to be frustrated in his need to succeed or was he able to overcome it in some way? Of course physical fitness is only one objective and how much importance is placed on it is a result of philosophy, but you should realize from this example that it is not only the student who is being evaluated but also, and perhaps primarily, it is the effectiveness of the instructor's program and methods which are reflected in student performance.

Movement skill is the core of our discipline. Sport and dance are our subject matter—we teach them, but perhaps more importantly, we teach through them. The teacher of English uses language and literature to help his students develop skills of communication, appreciation and response to the beauty of language as an art form. When English is taught in this manner it is not only a practical, in a sense vocational, course but it becomes one of the humanities. Movement skills also have their practical applications and they too may be art forms. It is not the subject matter which determines quality in teaching but rather it is the approach of the teacher and the scope of the program which will determine what the students may gain.

Not only would such a philosophy preclude a program consisting of the constant repetition of skills which have already been mastered but it would require the inclusion of a variety of activities which would encompass the full range of movement experiences available in our field. This challenge also presents arguments for homogeneous grouping in order to take our students to as high skill levels as possible.

Since motor ability does not appear to be a general quality but rather specific to the activity, grouping according to ability should be accomplished within the class and as specific activity units change. This involves preliminary skill testing in order to place students in, for example, beginning, intermediate or advanced basketball. The unit may then be taught at the two or three levels selected, thus eliminating the necessity for advanced skill students to repeat and for beginning skill students to compete outside of their ability range.

The arguments for a varied program include the challenge of learning new skills, the opportunity to acquire skills in lifetime sports activities, and the expansion of appreciations of movement forms. Although these arguments are worthy in themselves it might be necessary to present evidence to the school administrators to show that the students have acquired sufficient knowledge and skill in some activities and so by their elimination or limitation new activities may be started. Evaluation of present levels of student achievement could provide such evidence.

Research has indicated that for most effective learning, knowledge of results, and therefore progress, should be as immediate to the task as possible. Of course, in physical education activities results are frequently immediately observed (for either the ball goes through the basket or it does not) but improvement is not always so easily observed. When a student can see progress he is motivated to try harder even though he may still have a long way to go. The instructor also needs to measure student progress to determine the effectiveness of his methods. Of course a variety of methods is desirable since students learn in different ways, but teaching should always involve a constant process of evaluation. The teacher is encouraged to experiment with different methods of presentation but he needs to be able to determine whether or not they are superior to the old.

Grading is probably the least important purpose for which measurement is used, although the beginning teacher may give it primary importance. If the process of evaluation has resulted in a good program in which the students are properly classified and if progress is evident, then giving grades will be greatly simplified. Unhappiness with grades comes from the beginner who must compete with advanced students, the student with a disability for whom special objectives have not been set, the bored student to whom the grade is meaningless because he has learned nothing new, and the student who thought he was doing better than he was and did not find out until it was too late to try harder. When any instructor gives grades he must be able to explain and justify them in the light of objectives.

Evaluation in physical education may be accomplished by both subjective and objective means. We attempt to be as objective as possible in our determinations and we have devised instruments which assign quantitative values to the qualities being measured, but we also realize that some things do not lend themselves well to numerical assessment, that there are some qualities of humanness which may only be properly evaluated through human subjectivity. The instructor should be skilled in both objective and subjective evaluation for each has its part to play in the total evaluative process, and in most instances evaluation is accomplished through a combination of the two. For example: one might administer a battery of skill tests in assigning grades to specific skills in basketball, make use of rating scales (involving subjective judgments) in assessing game play and teamwork, and use subjective evaluations of the quality of movement in performance. One might add to this a written test utilizing both objectively constructed and subjectively evaluated (essay) questions. The final evaluation would then be the result of all of these methods combined according to their merits.

The following chapters are devoted to presentation of many of the evaluative tools in physical education, to discussion of their strengths and limitations, and to guidance in development of a philosophy of evaluation. The necessary foundation for an effective program of evaluation is a well-thought-out philosophy of physical education. When we know what we want to accomplish we know what needs to be evaluated. Evaluation is not an end to be sought but merely a means of providing a program which will meet the needs of our students.

Tests in
Physical Education

Test Selection

The instructor, having determined his philosophy and objectives of physical education will be ready to plan his evaluation program. The first step is to learn how to select good testing instruments.

There are many tests designed to measure the qualities involved in our objectives, and choosing which tests to use necessitates some thought. First of all the test should measure something which is considered important in our objectives. We should not test just for the sake of testing no matter how impressive it might look to the uninformed. The program will determine which qualities should be measured. Secondly we need to determine if the test which is selected is feasible for use in the situation. Will it take too much time to administer considering its importance to the program? Are the necessary equipment and facilities available? A test should be valid and reliable; it should really measure what it purports to measure (*validity*) and it should be consistent—if given again to the same group under exactly the same circumstance it should provide virtually the same results (*reliability*). No test will measure all of the qualities involved in an activity. A score for free-throw shooting in basketball, for instance, will not represent the student's ability to play the game. It will indicate a small part of that ability, and scores on a combination of such parts will, when considered together, give a better picture of the student's ability than will single measures. This ability of a test or test battery to measure and indicate the total quality is *validity*. Although a test of free throwing is a valid test of free throwing ability, the validity we are seeking is the relationship of a test to the overall quality being investigated, in this example, basketball playing ability.

Reliability is an indication of how flaw-proof a test may be. If there are ambiguities in the test or testing procedure the same person might do well one day and poorly the next. Luck may enter in, or conditions may interfere with the test's ability to measure performance and if this is the case the test is not very reliable. Of course a person changes from day to day but a reliable test will rank members of the class in approximately the same order if given again shortly after the first administration. Validity and reliability coefficients are presented for good tests, and being able to interpret these properly is important, for if an invalid test is used it will not measure the desired quality, and if a test has a low validity the instructor must take that into consideration when weighing the results derived from it in his evaluation. Validities and reliabilities are reported in the form of coefficients of correlation. We will discuss correlation coefficients and their meaning in a later section but a word here on what a good correlation is might be helpful.

Correlation is reported in decimals between plus one (+1.00) and minus one (-1.00). A perfect relationship between two sets of scores exists when the student with the highest score on the first test also scores highest on the second test, and the same situation is true of every student down to the student who scores poorest on both the first test and the second test. Such a perfect relationship illustrates a correlation of +1.00.

Inversely, should the highest scorer on the first test score lowest on the second, with each student achieving an equivalent opposite score, the perfect correlation in this case would be -1.00. When a good score on one test is recorded positively, as inches in the broad jump, and a good score on the second test is a low score, as seconds in the 50-yard dash, a negative correlation between these would actually represent a positive relationship.

If a test is *reliable,* consistent, and without flaws in administration, its reliability or *r* should equal .90 or above. Because of individual idiosyncracies, a headache or a quarrel with the girl friend, any one student might score well one day and poorly the next. The student himself may be inconsistent. These individual quirks might balance each other to some extent (as far as *group* records are concerned); even so it is not likely that a perfect correlation will ever be achieved. A high reliability is most important when judgments about individuals are to be made.

Validity is an entirely different situation. Since no one skill test can measure the total function of a game, validity coefficients will necessarily be lower than those of reliability. An example of a method of determining validity is to compare a student's ranking in a round-robin singles tennis tournament with his score on a tennis skill test. Presumably the best player in the class will win the tournament and should score highest on the skill test. Of course there are other factors to be considered in tournament play, but a test may be validated in this way.

A good validity coefficient on a skill test ranges upward from .60, with most falling in the .70's and a few exceptional tests with validities in the .80's.

You might ask what these decimals represent in terms of percentage of relationship. This can be determined by squaring the coefficient and treating the resulting number as a percentage. For example, a correlation of .50 is equivalent to a 25% relationship, .80 to 64%, and .90 to 81%. It is plain then that a validity of .70 which is fairly good, still only represents a relationship of 49% between the test and the activity.

When selecting a test it is necessary to consider these factors and weigh the test according to its predictive ability. It is fruitless to use an unreliable and invalid test.

It is not the purpose of this book to provide a comprehensive list of tests commonly used in physical education. You are referred to the many texts on measurement in physical education for a more comprehensive listing. The tests selected for presentation here are chosen for their ease of administration in terms of time and equipment needed, and for their scientific authenticity.

Strength

Strength is the most objective indication of general fitness since it is affected by physical, and to some extent, emotional difficulties, and since it lends itself to accurate measurement. Maintenance of strength acts as a preventative to certain health-related conditions such as coronary heart disease, diabetes, tension, and chronic fatigue. Strength should be maintained at a level above that necessary for accomplishing one's daily chores in order to provide for emergencies and effective use of leisure time.

The major difficulty in strength testing is that it usually requires specialized equipment not readily available to the public school teacher of physical education. Since strength is a factor in almost every test of fitness, motor ability, and skill it *is* being measured, at least indirectly, when these things are measured. We shall not, therefore, attempt to describe specific strength testing devices here, but you are referred to the bibliography should you wish to investigate further.

STRENGTH TESTS*

Three different test items are used to measure strength, depending upon the grade level and the sex of the pupil.

For Boys and Girls, Grades 4 Through 6

The modified pushup is the test item used to measure strength for boys and girls, grades 4 through 6.

a. Equipment and Testing Station

  1. Standard stall bar bench (11 by 21 by 14 inches)

  2. Mat

Place a standard stall bar bench on a mat near a flat wall surface.

b. Testing Procedure and Scoring

The pupil takes a standing position on the mat between the wall and the stall bar bench with his back to the wall. The pupil then leans forward, grasps the outer edges of the bench at the nearest corners and assumes the front leaning rest position, moving his feet back until both feet are flat against the wall. The body and arms must form a right angle (Figure 2.1). The bench should be placed at a

---

*State of New York, *The New York State Physical Fitness Test: A Manual For Teachers of Physical Education,* Albany, N.Y.: Division of Health, Physical Education, and Recreation, New York State Education Department, 1958. Adapted by permission of The State Department of Education.

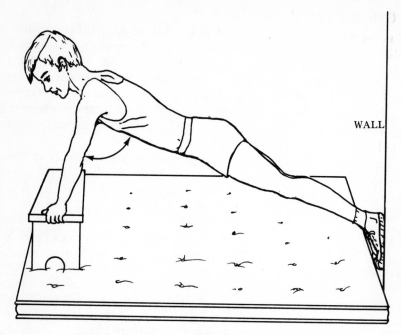

Figure 2.1. Strength Testing Position for Boys and Girls.

distance from the wall that is appropriate to the height of the pupil. Also, the smaller child may find it necessary to grasp the outer edges of the narrow dimensions of the bench if this width more closely approximates the width of the shoulders.

The pupil bends his arms until his upper chest lightly touches the near edge of the stall bar bench. He then pushes to a straight arm position. The pupil performs the pushup in this manner as many times as possible. The movement may be fast or slow, but there may be no rest between moves. The body must be held straight and the heels must remain in contact with the wall. In no case is the pupil permitted to raise or lower the hips out of line with the shoulders and feet.

Count one point for each complete pushup. If the body sways or arches, or if the pupil does not go down to the prescribed position or does not raise the body until the forearms are completely extended, the movement does not count. When the pupil is finished, record the total number of pushups on the Pupil Scorecard as the raw score. No half-pushups are counted. For safety, and for promoting confidence, the scorer should keep one hand lightly in contact with the arm of the pupil. He should also brace the bench if necessary.

For Girls, Grades 7 Through 12

The modified pullup is the test item used to measure strength for girls in grades 7 through 12.

a. Equipment and Testing Station

1. Standard horizontal bar or horizontal ladder

   (Note: If neither of these is available, a strong hardwood house ladder can be used)

2. Mat

Adjust the horizontal bar so that it is stabilized in the position where the girl can grasp the bar at a height even with the bottom of her sternum (breast bone). Provide appropriate matting under the equipment. If a ladder is used, it should be fastened securely to a rigid support such as the basketball backboard supports. The ladder should form an angle of about 45 degrees with the floor.

b. Testing Procedure and Scoring

From a standing position, the girl grasps the bar with the palms upward and slides the feet under the bar until the legs and the trunk are completely extended and until the arms form an angle of 90 degrees with the chest. The weight of the body should rest on the heels. The line of the body should form an angle of approximately 45 degrees with the floor line. The scorer should place the foot sidewise under the insteps of the pupil to prevent the feet from sliding on the mat (Figure 2.2).

The girl then pulls her body upward to the bar until her arms are completely bent and her chest touches the bar. The girl performs the pullups as many times as possible in this manner. The movement may be fast or slow, but there may be no rest between moves. Each time the girl must extend her arms completely.

Each pullup counts one point. If the hips sag or rise during the performance, the motion does not count. When the girl is finished, enter the number of complete pullups on the Pupil Scorecard as the raw score. No half-pullups are counted.

For Boys, Grades 7 Through 12

Full chinning or pullup is the test item used to measure strength for boys in grades 7 through 12.

a. Equipment and Testing Station

1. Standard horizontal bar

2. Mat

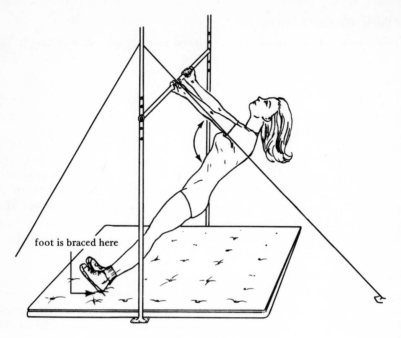

foot is braced here

Figure 2.2. Strength Testing Position for Girls.

Adjust the horizontal bar high enough so that the tallest boy may hang fully extended without touching the floor with his toes. Provide appropriate matting under the equipment.

b. Testing Procedure and Scoring

The pupil assumes as a starting position, a still hang; at full extension with an underhand or reverse grip, palms toward the face.

From this position, the pupil flexes his arms and pulls his body up to the bar until his arms are completely bent and his chin is level with the bar (Figure 2.3) and then lets himself down until his arms are fully extended. The boy chins himself in this manner as many times as possible. The movement may be fast or slow, but there may be no rest between moves. Each time he must lower himself all the way.

Each complete pullup counts one point. The feet may be together or apart, but no swinging or kicking is allowed when executing the chin. When the pupil is finished, enter the number of complete chins on the Pupil Scorecard as the raw score. No half chins are counted.

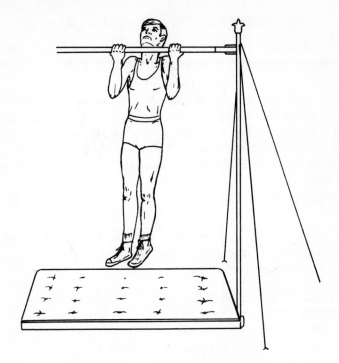

Figure 2.3. Strength Testing Position for Boys.

Endurance

The ability of the circulatory system to adjust to work would provide an effective indicator of condition if it were not subject to the influence of several extraneous variables (emotion, prior activity, eating) making its measurement not too reliable. Research on athletes and non-athletes has indicated some interesting facts however: Athletes have slower pulse rates, larger minute and stroke volumes, and pulse rates return to normal faster than non-athletes. The athlete's heart is more efficient.

Cardiovascular condition is usually determined by measuring the consumption of oxygen during a set time while a specific work load is accomplished. To do this requires elaborate equipment; however, the Harvard Step Test serves as a fairly indicative measure. Karpovich and Associates developed a rapid form of the Harvard Step Test which correlates very well with the form originally developed by Brouha.[10]

THE HARVARD STEP—UP TEST (rapid form)*

This test consists in measuring the endurance in stepping up and down on a bench 20 inches high and the pulse reaction to this exercise.

1. A subject steps up and down on a 20-inch bench at the rate of thirty complete steps per minute as long as he can, but not in excess of five minutes. Stepping up and down is done so that the lead foot may be alternated. The cadence of 120 counts per minute may be maintained by watching the swinging of a 39-inch-long pendulum.

2. Immediately after the test, the subject is seated and his pulse is taken.

The "rapid" form consists of taking the pulse count only once—from one minute to one minute and thirty seconds after the exercise. The score is obtained from the formula:

$$\text{Index of Fitness} = \frac{\text{Time of stepping in seconds} \times 100}{5.5 \text{ pulse count}}$$

The interpretation of scores is as follows:

Below 50 = Poor

50-80 = Average

Above 80 = Good.

Computations for the "rapid" form test may be avoided by the use of Table 2.1 shown on the opposite page.

Physical Fitness

The most commonly used test of physical fitness is that published by the AAHPER. This seven item test involves two races, (50-yard dash and the 600-yard run-walk); one throwing test (softball throw for distance); one arm-strength test (pullups or flex-arm hang); one trunk strength test (sit-ups); one test of power (standing broad jump); and one test of speed and agility (shuttle run).

---

*Karpovich, Peter V., *Physiology of Muscular Activity,* 6th Edition. W.B. Saunders Company. Used by permission of the author and publishers.

Table 1. Scoring Table for Harvard Step-Up Test (Rapid Form).

INSTRUCTIONS: (1) Find the appropriate line for duration of effort; (2) then find the appropriate column for the pulse count; (3) read off the score where the line and column intersect; and (4) interpret according to the scale given below.

Duration of Effort	Heart Beats from 1 Minute to 1 1/2 Minutes in Recovery										
	40–44	45–49	50–54	55–59	60–64	65–69	70–74	75–79	80–84	85–89	90–over
0′ - 29″	5	5	5	5	5	5	5	5	5	5	5
0′30″-0′59″	20	15	15	15	15	10	10	10	10	10	10
1′ 0″-1′29″	30	30	25	25	20	20	20	20	15	15	15
1′30″-1′59″	45	40	40	35	30	30	25	25	25	20	20
2′ 0″-2′29″	60	50	45	45	40	35	35	30	30	30	25
2′30″-2′59″	70	65	60	55	50	45	40	40	35	35	35
3′ 0″-3′29″	85	75	70	60	55	55	50	45	45	40	40
3′30″-3′59″	100	85	80	70	65	60	55	55	50	45	45
4′ 0″-4′29″	110	100	90	80	75	70	65	60	55	55	50
4′30″-4′59″	125	110	100	90	85	75	70	65	60	60	55
5′	130	115	105	95	90	80	75	70	65	65	60

Below 50 = Poor general physical fitness.
50–80 = Average general physical fitness.
Above 80 = Good general physical fitness.
Score of 75 accepted as minimum for
"good" condition.

This battery is designed to measure several components of physical fitness—strength, power, endurance, and flexibility. National norms have been established and reported in terms of percentiles. An evaluation of a student's physical fitness must be made in terms of all of the tests administered individually and as a battery. Should a student score well below the norm on any or all of the tests it would be anticipated that he would not be capable of performing up to his potential in physical activities; and because academic performance is related to physical condition, his low fitness probably would have a detrimental effect on all aspects of his school life. A program designed to condition him and raise his fitness level would be beneficial.

AAHPER FITNESS TESTS*

Pull-up

BOYS

Equipment

A metal or wooden bar approximately 1 1/2 inches in diameter is preferred. A doorway gym bar can be used, and, if no regular equipment is available, a piece of pipe or even the rungs of a ladder can also serve the purpose.

Description

The bar should be high enough so that the pupil can hang with his arms and legs fully extended and his feet free of the floor. He should use the overhand grasp (Figure 2.4). After assuming the hanging position, the pupil raises his body by his arms until his chin can be placed over the bar and then lowers his body to a full hang as in the starting position. The exercise is repeated as many times as possible.

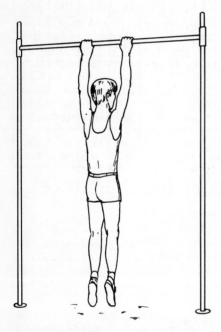

Figure 2.4. Starting Position for Pull-up.

Rules

1. Allow one trial unless it is obvious that the pupil has not had a fair chance.
2. The body must not swing during the execution of the movement. The pull must in no way be a snap movement. If the pupil starts swinging, check this by holding your extended arm across the front of the thighs.
3. The knees must not be raised and kicking of the legs is not permitted.

Scoring

Record the number of completed pull-ups to the nearest whole number.

*AAHPER, *Youth Fitness Test Manual,* Washington, D.C.: American Association for Health Physical Education, and Recreation. (1201 16th Street, N.W. Washington, D.C.) 1965. Used by permission of the AAHPER.

Flexed-Arm Hang

1

GIRLS

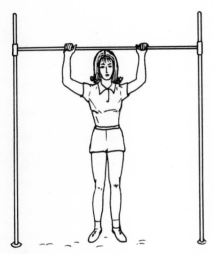

Figure 2.5. Starting Position for Flexed-Arm Hang.

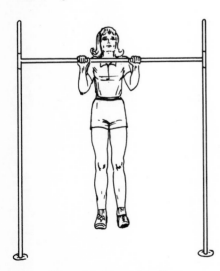

Figure 2.6. Flexed-Arm Hang.

Equipment

A horizontal bar approximately 1 1/2 inches in diameter is preferred. A doorway gym bar can be used; if no regular equipment is available, a piece of pipe can serve the purpose. A stop watch is needed.

Description

The height of the bar should be adjusted so it is approximately equal to the pupil's standing height. The pupil should use an overhand grasp (Figure 2.5). With the assistance of two spotters, one in front and one in back of pupil, the pupil raises her body off the floor to a position where the chin is above the bar, the elbows are flexed, and the chest is close to the bar (Figure 2.6). The pupil holds this position as long as possible.

Rules

1. The stop watch is started as soon as the subject takes the hanging position.
2. The watch is stopped when (a) pupil's chin touches the bar, (b) pupil's head tilts backwards to keep chin above the bar, (c) pupil's chin falls below the level of the bar.

Scoring

Record in seconds to the nearest second the length of time the subject holds the hanging position.

2

Sit-up

BOYS AND GIRLS

Equipment

Mat or floor.

Description

The pupil lies on his back, either on the floor or on a mat, with legs extended and feet about two feet apart. His hands are placed on the back of the neck with the fingers interlaced. Elbows are retracted. A partner holds the ankles down, the heels being in contact with the mat or floor at all times (Figure 2.7).

The pupil sits up, turning the trunk to the left and touching the right elbow to the left knee, returns to starting position, then sits up turning the trunk to the right and touching the left elbow to the right knee. The exercise is repeated, alternating sides (Figure 2.8).

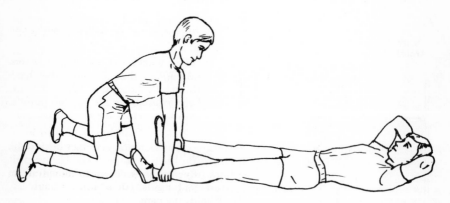

Figure 2.7. Starting Position for Sit-up.

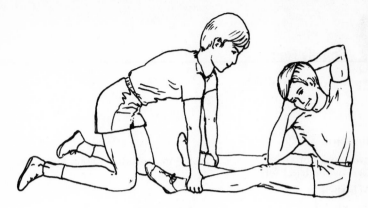

Figure 2.8. Sit-up.

Rules

1. The fingers must remain in contact behind the neck throughout the exercise.

2. The knees must be on the floor during the sit-up but may be slightly bent when touching elbow to knee.

3. The back should be rounded and the head and elbows brought forward when sitting up as a "curl" up.

4. When returning to starting position, elbows must be flat on the mat before sitting up again.

Scoring

One point is given for each complete movement of touching elbow to knee. No score should be counted if the fingertips do not maintain contact behind the head, if knees are bent when the pupil lies on his back or when he begins to sit up, or if the pupil pushes up off the floor from an elbow. The maximum limit in terms of number of sit-ups shall be: 50 sit-ups for girls, 100 sit-ups for boys.

3 Shuttle Run

BOYS AND GIRLS

Equipment

Two blocks of wood, 2 in. x 2 in. x 4 in., and stop watch. Pupils should wear sneakers or run barefooted.

Description

Two parallel lines are marked on the floor 30 feet apart. The width of a regulation volleyball court serves as a suitable area. Place the blocks of wood behind one of the lines as indicated in Figure 2.9. The pupil starts from behind the other line. On the signal "Ready? Go!," the pupil runs to the blocks, picks one up, runs back to the starting line and *places* the block behind the line; he then runs back and picks up the second block which he carries back across the starting line. If the scorer has two stop watches or one with a split-second timer, it is preferable to have two people running at the same time. To eliminate the necessity of returning the blocks after each race, start the races alternately, first from behind one line and then from behind the other.

Rules

Allow two trials with some rest between.

Scoring

Record the better of the two trials to the nearest tenth of a second.

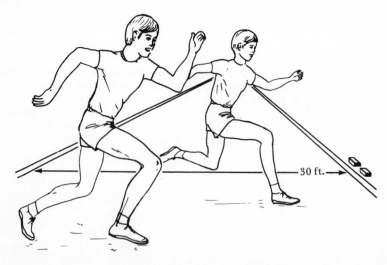

Figure 2.9. Starting the Shuttle Run.

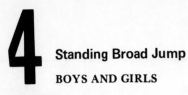

Standing Broad Jump

BOYS AND GIRLS

Equipment

Mat, floor, or outdoor jumping pit, and tape measure.

Description

Pupil stands as indicated in Figure 2.10, with the feet several inches apart and the toes just behind the take-off line. Preparatory to jumping, the pupil swings the arms backward and bends the knees. The jump is accomplished by simultaneously extending the knees and swinging forward the arms.

Rules

1. Allow three trials.
2. Measure from the take-off line to the heel or other part of the body that touches the floor nearest the take-off line (Figure 2.10).
3. When the test is given indoors, it is convenient to tape the tape measure to the floor at right angles to the take-off line and have the pupils jump along the tape. The scorer stands to the side and observes the mark to the nearest inch.

Scoring

Record the best of the three trials in feet and inches to the nearest inch.

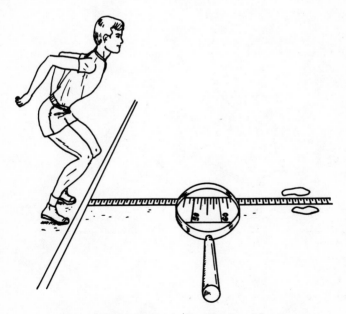

Figure 2.10. Measuring the Standing Broad Jump.

5 50-Yard Dash

BOYS AND GIRLS

Equipment

Two stop watches or one with a split-second timer.

Description

It is preferable to administer this test to two pupils at a time. Have both take positions behind the starting line. The starter will use the commands "Are you ready?" and "Go!" The latter will be accompanied by a downward sweep of the starter's arm to give the timer a visual signal.

Rules

The score is the amount of time between the starter's signal and the instant the pupil crosses the finish line.

Scoring

Record in seconds to the nearest tenth of a second.

6

Softball Throw for Distance

BOYS AND GIRLS

Equipment
Softball (12-inch), small metal or wooden stakes, and tape measure.

Description
A football field marked in conventional fashion (five-yard intervals) makes an ideal area for this test. If this is not available, it is suggested that lines be drawn parallel to the restraining line, five yards apart. The pupil throws the ball while remaining within two parallel lines, six feet apart (Figure 2.11). Mark the point of landing with one of the small stakes. If his second or third throw is farther, move the stake accordingly so that, after three throws, the stake is at the point of the pupil's best throw. It was found expedient to have the pupil jog out to his stake and stand there; and then, after five pupils have completed their throws, the measurements were taken. By having the pupil at his particular stake, there is little danger of recording the wrong score.

Rules
1. Only an overhand throw may be used.
2. Three throws are allowed.
3. The distance recorded is the distance measured at right angles from the point of landing to the restraining line (Figure 2.11).

Scoring
Record the best of the three trials to the nearest foot.

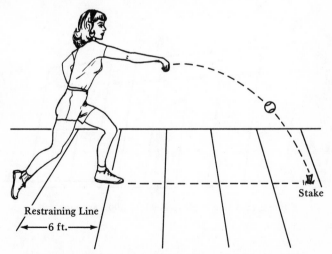

Restraining Line

←—6 ft.—→

Stake

Figure 2.11. Measuring the Softball Throw for Distance. Wherever Ball Lands, Measure Distance Perpendicular to Starting Line.

600-Yard Run-Walk

7

BOYS AND GIRLS

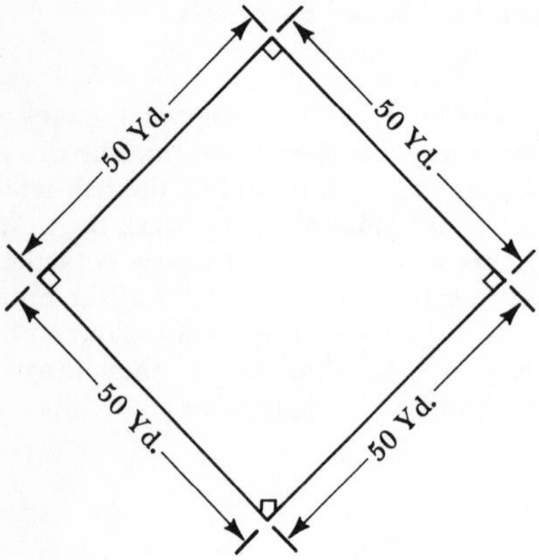

Equipment

Track or area marked according to Figure 2.13 and stop watch.

Description

Pupil uses a standing start. At the signal "Ready? Go!" the pupil starts running the 600-yard distance. The running may be interspersed with walking. It is possible to have a dozen pupils run at one time by having the pupils pair off before the start of the event. Then each pupil listens for and remembers his partner's time as the latter crosses the finish. The timer merely calls out the times as the pupils cross the finish.

Rules

Walking is permitted, but the object is to cover the distance in the shortest possible time.

Scoring

Record in minutes and seconds.

Figure 2.12. Using Any Open Area for 600-Yard Run-Walk.

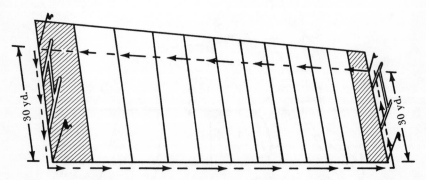

Figure 2.13. Using Football Field for 600-Yard Run-Walk.

Table 2.2. Flexed-Arm Hang For Girls
Percentile Scores Based on Age/Test Scores in Seconds

Percen-tile	Age								Percen-tile
	10	11	12	13	14	15	16	17	
100th	66	79	64	80	60	74	74	76	100th
95th	31	35	30	30	30	33	37	31	95th
90th	24	25	23	21	22	22	26	25	90th
85th	21	20	19	18	19	18	19	19	85th
80th	18	17	15	15	16	16	16	16	80th
75th	15	16	13	13	13	14	14	14	75th
70th	13	13	11	12	11	13	12	12	70th
65th	11	11	10	10	10	11	10	11	65th
60th	10	10	8	9	9	10	9	10	60th
55th	9	9	8	8	8	8	8	9	55th
50th	7	8	6	7	7	8	7	8	50th
45th	6	6	6	6	6	6	6	7	45th
40th	6	5	5	5	5	6	5	6	40th
35th	5	4	4	4	4	4	4	4	35th
30th	4	4	3	3	3	3	3	4	30th
25th	3	3	2	2	2	2	2	3	25th
20th	2	2	1	2	1	1	1	2	20th
15th	2	1	0	1	1	0	1	0	15th
10th	1	0	0	0	0	0	0	0	10th
5th	0	0	0	0	0	0	0	0	5th
0	0	0	0	0	0	0	0	0	0

Table 2.3. Sit-Ups For Girls
Percentile Scores Based on Age

Percen-tile	Age								Percen-tile
	10	11	12	13	14	15	16	17	
100th	50	50	50	50	50	50	50	50	100th
95th	50	50	50	50	49	37	40	42	95th
90th	50	50	39	36	34	31	32	37	90th
85th	40	40	34	30	30	28	30	30	85th
80th	33	34	30	30	28	26	27	25	80th
75th	30	30	29	27	25	24	25	24	75th
70th	27	29	25	25	24	22	24	23	70th
65th	24	26	24	23	22	20	22	21	65th
60th	22	25	22	21	20	20	21	20	60th
55th	20	23	21	20	20	19	20	18	55th
50th	19	20	20	20	18	18	19	16	50th
45th	17	20	18	19	17	16	18	15	45th
40th	15	18	17	17	15	15	16	15	40th
35th	14	16	15	16	14	14	15	14	35th
30th	12	15	13	15	12	13	13	12	30th
25th	11	13	12	13	11	11	12	11	25th
20th	10	11	10	12	10	10	11	9	20th
15th	8	10	10	10	8	8	10	8	15th
10th	6	8	7	8	6	6	8	6	10th
5th	4	5	5	5	4	4	4	3	5th
0	0	0	0	0	0	0	0	0	0

Table 2.4 Shuttle Run For Girls
Percentile Scores Based on Age/Test Scores in Seconds and Tenths

Percen-tile	Age								Percen-tile
	10	11	12	13	14	15	16	17	
100th	8.5	8.8	9.0	8.3	9.0	8.0	8.3	9.0	100th
95th	10.0	10.0	10.0	10.0	10.0	10.0	10.0	10.0	95th
90th	10.5	10.2	10.2	10.2	10.3	10.3	10.2	10.3	90th
85th	10.8	10.6	10.5	10.5	10.4	10.5	10.4	10.4	85th
80th	11.0	10.9	10.8	10.6	10.5	10.7	10.6	10.5	80th
75th	11.0	11.0	10.9	10.8	10.6	10.9	10.8	10.6	75th
70th	11.1	11.0	11.0	11.0	10.8	11.0	10.9	10.8	70th
65th	11.4	11.2	11.2	11.0	10.9	11.0	11.0	11.0	65th
60th	11.5	11.4	11.3	11.1	11.0	11.1	11.0	11.0	60th
55th	11.8	11.6	11.5	11.3	11.1	11.2	11.2	11.1	55th
50th	11.9	11.7	11.6	11.4	11.3	11.3	11.2	11.2	50th
45th	12.0	11.8	11.8	11.6	11.4	11.5	11.4	11.4	45th
40th	12.0	12.0	11.9	11.8	11.5	11.6	11.5	11.5	40th
35th	12.1	12.0	12.0	12.0	11.7	11.8	11.8	11.6	35th
30th	12.4	12.1	12.1	12.0	12.0	11.9	12.0	11.8	30th
25th	12.6	12.4	12.3	12.2	12.0	12.0	12.0	12.0	25th
20th	12.8	12.6	12.5	12.5	12.3	12.3	12.2	12.0	20th
15th	13.0	13.0	12.9	13.0	12.6	12.5	12.5	12.3	15th
10th	13.1	13.4	13.2	13.3	13.1	13.0	13.0	13.0	10th
5th	14.0	14.1	13.9	14.0	13.9	13.5	13.9	13.8	5th
0	16.6	18.5	19.8	18.5	17.6	16.0	17.6	10.0	0

Table 2.5. Standing Broad Jump For Girls
Percentile Scores Based on Age

Percen-tile	Age								Percen-tile
	10	11	12	13	14	15	16	17	
100th	6' 2"	7' 1"	6'11"	6' 8"	6'11"	7' 0"	7' 2"	7' 0"	100th
95th	5' 4"	5' 7"	5' 8"	5' 9"	6' 0"	6' 2"	6' 5"	6' 6"	95th
90th	5' 1"	5' 4"	5' 6"	5' 7"	5' 9"	6' 0"	6' 0"	6' 2"	90th
85th	4'11"	5' 2"	5' 3"	5' 5"	5' 7"	5' 9"	5'11"	6' 0"	85th
80th	4'10"	5' 0"	5' 2"	5' 4"	5' 6"	5' 6"	5' 8"	5'10"	80th
75th	4' 8"	4'11"	5' 0"	5' 2"	5' 4"	5' 4"	5' 6"	5' 8"	75th
70th	4' 7"	4'10"	4'11"	5' 1"	5' 2"	5' 3"	5' 5"	5' 7"	70th
65th	4' 6"	4' 8"	4'10"	5' 0"	5' 1"	5' 2"	5' 3"	5' 5"	65th
60th	4' 5"	4' 8"	4' 9"	4'11"	5' 0"	5' 0"	5' 2"	5' 3"	60th
55th	4' 4"	4' 6"	4' 7"	4' 9"	4'10"	5' 0"	5' 1"	5' 2"	55th
50th	4' 3"	4' 6"	4' 6"	4' 8"	4' 9"	4'10"	5' 0"	5' 0"	50th
45th	4' 2"	4' 4"	4' 6"	4' 7"	4' 8"	4' 9"	4'11"	5' 0"	45th
40th	4' 1"	4' 3"	4' 5"	4' 6"	4' 7"	4' 8"	4'10"	4'10"	40th
35th	4' 0"	4' 2"	4' 3"	4' 5"	4' 6"	4' 7"	4' 9"	4' 8"	35th
30th	3'10"	4' 0"	4' 2"	4' 4"	4' 5"	4' 5"	4' 8"	4' 7"	30th
25th	3' 9"	3'11"	4' 1"	4' 3"	4' 4"	4' 4"	4' 6"	4' 6"	25th
20th	3' 8"	3'10"	4' 0"	4' 2"	4' 2"	4' 3"	4' 4"	4' 4"	20th
15th	3' 6"	3' 8"	3'10"	3'11"	4' 0"	4' 1"	4' 3"	4' 2"	15th
10th	3' 4"	3' 6"	3' 9"	3' 9"	3'10"	4' 0"	4' 0"	4' 0"	10th
5th	3' 2"	3' 3"	3' 5"	3' 6"	3' 6"	3' 8"	3'10"	3' 7"	5th
0	2' 5"	2' 5"	2' 9"	2' 7"	2' 3"	3' 0"	2' 6"	3' 1"	0

Table 2.6. 50-Yard Dash For Girls
Percentile Scores Based on
Age/Test Scores in Seconds and Tenths

Percen-tile	Age								Percen-tile
	10	11	12	13	14	15	16	17	
100th	6.0	6.0	5.9	6.0	6.0	6.4	6.0	6.4	100th
95th	7.0	7.0	7.0	7.0	7.0	7.1	7.0	7.1	95th
90th	7.3	7.4	7.3	7.3	7.2	7.3	7.3	7.3	90th
85th	7.5	7.6	7.5	7.5	7.4	7.5	7.5	7.5	85th
80th	7.7	7.7	7.6	7.6	7.5	7.6	7.5	7.6	80th
75th	7.9	7.9	7.8	7.7	7.6	7.7	7.7	7.8	75th
70th	8.0	8.0	7.9	7.8	7.7	7.8	7.9	7.9	70th
65th	8.1	8.0	8.0	7.9	7.8	7.9	8.0	8.0	65th
60th	8.2	8.1	8.0	8.0	7.9	8.0	8.0	8.0	60th
55th	8.4	8.2	8.1	8.0	8.0	8.0	8.1	8.1	55th
50th	8.5	8.4	8.2	8.1	8.0	8.1	8.3	8.2	50th
45th	8.6	8.5	8.3	8.2	8.2	8.2	8.4	8.3	45th
40th	8.8	8.5	8.4	8.4	8.3	8.3	8.5	8.5	40th
35th	8.9	8.6	8.5	8.5	8.5	8.4	8.6	8.6	35th
30th	9.0	8.8	8.7	8.6	8.6	8.6	8.8	8.8	30th
25th	9.0	9.0	8.9	8.8	8.9	8.8	9.0	9.0	25th
20th	9.2	9.0	9.0	9.0	9.0	9.0	9.0	9.0	20th
15th	9.4	9.2	9.2	9.2	9.2	9.0	9.2	9.1	15th
10th	9.6	9.6	9.5	9.5	9.5	9.5	9.9	9.5	10th
5th	10.0	10.0	10.0	10.2	10.4	10.0	10.5	10.4	5th
0	14.0	13.0	13.0	15.7	16.0	18.0	17.0	12.0	0

Table 2.7. Softball Throw For Girls
Percentile Scores Based on Age

Percen-tile	Age								Percen-tile
	10	11	12	13	14	15	16	17	
100th	108	149	152	187	193	170	169	169	100th
95th	69	88	94	106	112	117	120	120	95th
90th	63	78	86	100	102	107	110	112	90th
85th	58	72	82	92	94	99	102	108	85th
80th	56	68	78	88	89	94	99	102	80th
75th	53	65	74	84	85	89	94	97	75th
70th	50	62	70	80	82	86	90	93	70th
65th	47	59	68	77	78	84	87	90	65th
60th	45	56	65	75	75	80	84	86	60th
55th	43	54	62	72	72	78	80	84	55th
50th	41	51	60	69	70	74	76	79	50th
45th	40	50	57	66	67	70	75	75	45th
40th	38	48	55	63	64	67	71	72	40th
35th	37	45	52	60	62	65	69	69	35th
30th	35	43	50	58	59	61	65	66	30th
25th	33	41	48	54	56	58	61	63	25th
20th	31	38	45	50	54	56	59	60	20th
15th	30	36	42	48	50	52	54	54	15th
10th	28	33	40	44	45	48	49	49	10th
5th	26	30	35	39	33	42	44	43	5th
0	13	16	21	19	18	10	28	30	0

Table 2.8. 600-Yard Run-Walk For Girls
Percentile Scores Based on
Age/Test Scores in Minutes and Seconds

Percen-tile	Age								Percen-tile
	10	11	12	13	14	15	16	17	
100th	1'42"	1'40"	1'39"	1'40"	1'45"	1'40"	1'50"	1'54"	100th
95th	2' 5"	2'13"	2'14"	2'12"	2' 9"	2' 9"	2'10"	2'11"	95th
90th	2'15"	2'19"	2'20"	2'19"	2'18"	2'18"	2'17"	2'22"	90th
85th	2'20"	2'24"	2'24"	2'25"	2'22"	2'23"	2'23"	2'27"	85th
80th	2'26"	2'28"	2'27"	2'29"	2'25"	2'26"	2'26"	2'31"	80th
75th	2'30"	2'32"	2'31"	2'33"	2'30"	2'28"	2'31"	2'34"	75th
70th	2'34"	2'36"	2'35"	2'37"	2'34"	2'34"	2'36"	2'37"	70th
65th	2'37"	2'39"	2'39"	2'40"	2'37"	2'36"	2'39"	2'42"	65th
60th	2'41"	2'43"	2'42"	2'44"	2'41"	2'40"	2'42"	2'46"	60th
55th	2'45"	2'47"	2'45"	2'47"	2'44"	2'43"	2'45"	2'49"	55th
50th	2'48"	2'49"	2'49"	2'52"	2'46"	2'46"	2'49"	2'51"	50th
45th	2'50"	2'53"	2'55"	2'56"	2'51"	2'49"	2'53"	2'57"	45th
40th	2'55"	2'59"	2'58"	3' 0"	2'55"	2'52"	2'56"	3' 0"	40th
35th	2'59"	3' 4"	3' 3"	3' 3"	3' 0"	2'56"	2'59"	3' 5"	35th
30th	3' 3"	3'10"	3' 7"	3' 9"	3' 6"	3' 0"	3' 1"	3'10"	30th
25th	3' 8"	3'15"	3'11"	3'15"	3'12"	3' 5"	3' 7"	3'16"	25th
20th	3'13"	3'22"	3'18"	3'20"	3'19"	3'10"	3'12"	3'22"	20th
15th	3'18"	3'30"	3'24"	3'30"	3'30"	3'18"	3'19"	3'29"	15th
10th	3'27"	3'41"	3'40"	3'49"	3'48"	3'28"	3'30"	3'41"	10th
5th	3'45"	3'59"	4' 0"	4'11"	4' 8"	3'56"	3'45"	3'56"	5th
0	4'47"	4'53"	5'10"	5'10"	5'50"	5'10"	5'52"	6'40"	0

Table 2.9. Pull-Ups For Boys
Percentile Scores Based on Age

Percen-tile	Age								Percen-tile
	10	11	12	13	14	15	16	17	
100th	12	11	20	14	15	20	18	16	100th
95th	6	6	7	8	10	10	13	12	95th
90th	5	5	6	7	8	9	11	11	90th
85th	4	4	5	6	7	8	10	10	85th
80th	3	4	4	5	6	7	9	10	80th
75th	2	3	4	4	5	6	8	9	75th
70th	2	2	3	4	5	5	7	8	70th
65th	2	2	3	4	4	5	7	7	65th
60th	1	2	2	3	4	5	6	7	60th
55th	1	1	2	3	3	4	6	6	55th
50th	1	1	2	2	3	4	5	6	50th
45th	1	1	1	2	2	4	5	5	45th
40th	0	1	1	2	2	3	4	5	40th
35th	0	0	1	1	2	3	4	4	35th
30th	0	0	1	1	1	2	3	4	30th
25th	0	0	0	1	1	2	3	3	25th
20th	0	0	0	0	1	1	3	3	20th
15th	0	0	0	0	0	1	2	3	15th
10th	0	0	0	0	0	1	2	2	10th
5th	0	0	0	0	0	0	1	1	5th
0	0	0	0	0	0	0	0	0	0

Table 2.10. Sit-Ups For Boys
Percentile Scores Based on Age/Test Scores in Number of Sit-Ups

Percen-tile	Age								Percen-tile
	10	11	12	13	14	15	16	17	
100th	100	100	100	100	100	100	100	100	100th
95th	100	100	100	100	100	100	100	100	95th
90th	100	100	100	100	100	100	100	100	90th
85th	100	100	100	100	100	100	100	100	85th
80th	76	89	100	100	100	100	100	100	80th
75th	65	73	93	100	100	100	100	100	75th
70th	57	60	75	99	100	100	100	100	70th
65th	51	55	70	90	99	100	99	99	65th
60th	50	50	59	75	99	99	99	85	60th
55th	49	50	52	70	77	90	85	77	55th
50th	41	46	50	60	70	80	76	70	50th
45th	37	40	49	53	62	70	70	62	45th
40th	34	35	42	50	60	61	63	57	40th
35th	30	31	40	50	52	54	56	51	35th
30th	28	30	35	41	50	50	50	50	30th
25th	25	26	30	38	45	49	50	45	25th
20th	23	23	28	35	40	42	42	40	20th
15th	20	20	25	30	36	39	38	35	15th
10th	15	17	20	25	30	33	34	30	10th
5th	11	12	15	20	24	27	28	23	5th
0	1	0	0	1	6	5	10	8	0

Table 2.11. Shuttle Run For Boys
Percentile Scores Based on Age

Percen-tile	Age								Percen-tile
	10	11	12	13	14	15	16	17	
100th	8.7	9.2	9.0	8.1	8.1	8.0	8.2	8.5	100th
95th	10.3	10.4	10.0	9.7	9.4	9.3	9.1	9.0	95th
90th	10.8	10.6	10.2	10.0	9.8	9.5	9.3	9.2	90th
85th	11.0	10.9	10.4	10.2	9.9	9.8	9.4	9.3	85th
80th	11.2	11.0	10.5	10.3	10.0	10.0	9.5	9.5	80th
75th	11.4	11.2	10.8	10.5	10.2	10.0	9.6	9.6	75th
70th	11.6	11.3	10.9	10.6	10.2	10.1	9.8	9.8	70th
65th	11.7	11.5	11.0	10.7	10.4	10.2	10.0	10.0	65th
60th	11.9	11.6	11.1	10.8	10.5	10.4	10.0	10.0	60th
55th	12.0	11.7	11.2	11.0	10.6	10.5	10.2	10.1	55th
50th	12.1	11.8	11.4	11.0	10.8	10.6	10.3	10.3	50th
45th	12.2	12.0	11.5	11.3	10.9	10.7	10.4	10.5	45th
40th	12.3	12.0	11.7	11.5	11.0	10.9	10.5	10.6	40th
35th	12.5	12.2	11.9	11.6	11.1	11.0	10.7	10.8	35th
30th	12.6	12.4	12.0	11.8	11.2	11.2	10.9	10.9	30th
25th	12.9	12.5	12.3	12.0	11.4	11.3	11.0	11.1	25th
20th	13.0	12.8	12.5	12.3	11.5	11.5	11.2	11.3	20th
15th	13.4	13.0	12.7	12.5	11.8	11.7	11.5	11.5	15th
10th	13.7	13.5	13.2	13.0	12.0	12.0	12.0	12.0	10th
5th	14.3	14.0	14.0	13.2	12.5	12.9	12.6	12.5	5th
0	16.0	16.1	16.5	18.0	15.2	15.0	17.5	17.6	0

Table 2.12. Standing Broad Jump For Boys
Percentile Scores Based on Age/Test Scores in Feet and Inches

Percen-tile	Age								Percen-tile
	10	11	12	13	14	15	16	17	
100th	6' 8"	10' 0"	7'10"	8' 9"	8'11"	9' 2"	9' 1"	9' 8"	100th
95th	6' 1"	6' 3"	6' 6"	7' 2"	7' 9"	8' 0"	8' 5"	8' 6"	95th
90th	5'10"	6' 0"	6' 4"	6'11"	7' 5"	7' 9"	8' 1"	8' 3"	90th
85th	5' 8"	5'10"	6' 2"	6' 9"	7' 3"	7' 6"	7'11"	8' 1"	85th
80th	5' 7"	5' 9"	6' 1"	6' 7"	7' 0"	7' 6"	7' 9"	8' 0"	80th
75th	5' 6"	5' 7"	6' 0"	6' 5"	6'11"	7' 4"	7' 7"	7'10"	75th
70th	5' 5"	5' 6"	5'11"	6' 3"	6' 9"	7' 2"	7' 6"	7' 8"	70th
65th	5' 4"	5' 6"	5' 9"	6' 1"	6' 8"	7' 1"	7' 5"	7' 7"	65th
60th	5' 2"	5' 4"	5' 8"	6' 0"	6' 7"	7' 0"	7' 4"	7' 6"	60th
55th	5' 1"	5' 3"	5' 7"	5'11"	6' 6"	6'11"	7' 3"	7' 5"	55th
50th	5' 0"	5' 2"	5' 6"	5'10"	6' 4"	6' 9"	7' 1"	7' 3"	50th
45th	5' 0"	5' 1"	5' 5"	5' 9"	6' 3"	6' 8"	7' 0"	7' 2"	45th
40th	4'10"	5' 0"	5' 4"	5' 7"	6' 1"	6' 6"	6'11"	7' 0"	40th
35th	4'10"	4'11"	5' 2"	5' 6"	6' 0"	6' 6"	6' 9"	6'11"	35th
30th	4' 8"	4'10"	5' 1"	5' 5"	5'10"	6' 4"	6' 7"	6'10"	30th
25th	4' 6"	4' 8"	5' 0"	5' 3"	5' 8"	6' 3"	6' 6"	6' 8"	25th
20th	4' 5"	4' 7"	4'10"	5' 2"	5' 6"	6' 1"	6' 4"	6' 6"	20th
15th	4' 4"	4' 5"	4' 8"	5' 0"	5' 4"	5'10"	6' 1"	6' 4"	15th
10th	4' 3"	4' 2"	4' 5"	4' 9"	5' 2"	5' 7"	5'11"	6' 0"	10th
5th	4' 0"	4' 0"	4' 2"	4' 5"	4'11"	5' 4"	5' 6"	5' 8"	5th
0	2'10"	1' 8"	3' 0"	2' 9"	3' 8"	2'10"	2' 2"	3' 7"	0

Table 2.13. 50-Yard Dash For Boys
Percentile Scores Based on Age

Percen-tile	Age								Percen-tile
	10	11	12	13	14	15	16	17	
100th	6.5	6.1	6.0	5.8	5.6	5.5	5.4	5.4	100th
95th	7.6	7.3	7.0	6.5	6.5	6.2	6.1	6.0	95th
90th	7.9	7.5	7.2	6.9	6.8	6.4	6.2	6.1	90th
85th	8.0	7.7	7.4	7.0	6.9	6.5	6.3	6.2	85th
80th	8.1	7.9	7.5	7.2	7.0	6.7	6.4	6.3	80th
75th	8.3	8.0	7.6	7.3	7.1	6.8	6.5	6.4	75th
70th	8.4	8.1	7.8	7.4	7.2	6.9	6.6	6.5	70th
65th	8.5	8.2	7.9	7.5	7.3	7.0	6.7	6.6	65th
60th	8.6	8.3	8.0	7.6	7.3	7.0	6.8	6.6	60th
55th	8.7	8.4	8.0	7.7	7.4	7.1	6.9	6.7	55th
50th	8.8	8.5	8.0	7.8	7.5	7.1	7.0	6.8	50th
45th	9.0	8.6	8.2	7.9	7.6	7.2	7.0	6.9	45th
40th	9.0	8.7	8.3	8.0	7.7	7.3	7.0	7.0	40th
35th	9.2	8.8	8.4	8.0	7.8	7.4	7.1	7.0	35th
30th	9.3	8.9	8.5	8.2	7.9	7.5	7.2	7.1	30th
25th	9.4	9.0	8.6	8.3	8.0	7.6	7.3	7.2	25th
20th	9.6	9.1	8.8	8.5	8.1	7.8	7.4	7.3	20th
15th	9.7	9.4	9.0	8.6	8.2	8.0	7.6	7.5	15th
10th	10.0	9.7	9.2	9.0	8.5	8.0	7.8	7.6	10th
5th	10.8	10.2	9.6	9.3	8.8	8.5	8.0	7.9	5th
0	13.5	14.3	13.6	12.5	10.1	10.5	9.7	9.3	0

Table 2.14. Softball Throw For Boys
Percentile Scores Based on Age/Test Scores in Feet

Percen-tile	Age								Percen-tile
	10	11	12	13	14	15	16	17	
100th	175	205	207	245	246	250	271	291	100th
95th	138	151	165	195	208	221	238	249	95th
90th	127	141	156	183	195	210	222	235	90th
85th	122	136	150	175	187	204	213	226	85th
80th	118	129	145	168	181	198	207	218	80th
75th	114	126	141	163	176	192	201	213	75th
70th	109	121	136	157	172	189	197	207	70th
65th	105	119	133	152	168	184	194	203	65th
60th	102	115	129	147	165	180	189	198	60th
55th	98	113	124	142	160	175	185	195	55th
50th	96	111	120	140	155	171	180	190	50th
45th	93	108	119	135	150	167	175	185	45th
40th	91	105	115	131	146	165	172	180	40th
35th	89	101	112	128	141	160	168	176	35th
30th	84	98	110	125	138	156	165	171	30th
25th	81	94	106	120	133	152	160	163	25th
20th	78	90	103	115	127	147	153	155	20th
15th	73	85	97	110	122	141	147	150	15th
10th	69	78	92	101	112	135	141	141	10th
5th	60	70	76	88	102	123	127	117	5th
0	35	14	25	50	31	60	30	31	0

Table 2.15. 600-Yard Run-Walk For Boys
Percentile Scores Based on Age

Percen-tile	Age								Percen—tile
	10	11	12	13	14	15	16	17	
100th	1:45	1:39	1:45	1:40	1:30	1:23	1:30	1:25	100th
95th	2:45	2:02	2:05	2:00	1:50	1:43	1:40	1:36	95th
90th	2:23	2:15	2:12	2:05	1:56	1:50	1:45	1:44	90th
85th	2:27	2:21	2:16	2:10	2:02	1:55	1:48	1:48	85th
80th	2:30	2:24	2:19	2:13	2:05	1:59	1:51	1:51	80th
75th	2:34	2:27	2:22	2:15	2:08	2:01	1:54	1:54	75th
70th	2:38	2:31	2:26	2:18	2:11	2:05	1:56	1:55	70th
65th	2:41	2:34	2:29	2:21	2:13	2:07	1:59	1:58	65th
60th	2:45	2:37	2:32	2:25	2:18	2:09	2:00	2:00	60th
55th	2:48	2:40	2:35	2:27	2:20	2:10	2:03	2:02	55th
50th	2:51	2:43	2:39	2:29	2:22	2:14	2:05	2:04	50th
45th	2:55	2:47	2:42	2:32	2:25	2:17	2:07	2:06	45th
40th	2:58	2:50	2:46	2:36	2:30	2:20	2:10	2:09	40th
35th	3:03	2:56	2:50	2:40	2:34	2:24	2:12	2:14	35th
30th	3:06	3:01	2:56	2:44	2:37	2:28	2:16	2:17	30th
25th	3:10	3:07	3:02	2:50	2:44	2:31	2:23	2:22	25th
20th	3:15	3:12	3:06	2:57	2:52	2:25	2:30	2:26	20th
15th	3:23	3:20	3:17	3:02	3:00	2:42	2:36	2:35	15th
10th	3:36	3:29	3:33	3:15	3:14	2:55	2:41	2:44	10th
5th	3:48	3:48	3:50	3:39	3:33	3:16	3:02	3:05	5th
0	5:02	5:06	7:00	5:45	5:45	5:37	5:35	5:00	0

Table 2.16. Percentile Scores For College Women

Percentile	Modified Pull-Ups	Sit-Ups	Shuttle Run	St. Broad Jump	50-Yd. Dash	Softball Throw	Run-Walk 600-Yd.
100	40	50	7.5	7'10"	5.4	184	1:49
95	39	43	10.2	6'6"	7.3	115	2:19
90	38	35	10.5	6'3"	7.6	103	2:27
85	33	31	10.7	6'1"	7.7	96	2:32
80	30	29	10.9	5'11"	7.8	90	2:37
75	28	27	11.0	5'10"	7.9	86	2:41
70	26	25	11.1	5'8"	8.0	82	2:44
65	24	24	11.2	5'7"	8.1	79	2:48
60	22	22	11.3	5'6"	8.2	76	2:51
55	21	21	11.5	5'5"	8.3	73	2:54
50	20	20	11.6	5'4"	8.4	70	2:58
45	18	19	11.7	5'3"	8.6	67	3:01
40	17	18	11.9	5'2"	8.7	65	3:05
35	16	16	12.0	5'0"	8.8	62	3:08
30	15	15	12.1	4'11"	9.0	59	3:13
25	13	14	12.2	4'10"	9.1	57	3:18
20	12	13	12.4	4'8"	9.2	54	3:23
15	11	11	12.6	4'7"	9.4	51	3:29
10	9	9	12.9	4'5"	9.7	47	3:38
5	7	7	13.4	4'1"	10.1	42	3:53
0	0	0	17.3	2'3"	13.7	5	5:29

Table 2.17. Percentile Scores For College Men

Percentile	Pull-Ups	Sit-Ups	Shuttle Run	St. Broad Jump	50-Yd. Dash	Softball Throw	600-Yd. Run-Walk
100	20	100	8.3	9'6"	5.5	315	1:12
95	12	99	9.0	8'5"	6.1	239	1:35
90	10	97	9.1	8'2"	6.2	226	1:38
85	10	79	9.1	7'11"	6.3	217	1:40
80	9	68	9.2	7'10"	6.4	211	1:42
75	8	61	9.4	7'8"	6.5	206	1:44
70	8	58	9.5	7'7"	6.5	200	1:45
65	7	52	9.5	7'6"	6.6	196	1:47
60	7	51	9.6	7'5"	6.6	192	1:49
55	6	50	9.6	7'4"	6.7	188	1:50
50	6	47	9.7	7'3"	6.8	184	1:52
45	5	44	9.8	7'1"	6.8	180	1:53
40	5	41	9.9	7'0"	6.9	176	1:55
35	4	38	10.0	6'11"	7.0	171	1:57
30	4	36	10.0	6'10"	7.0	166	1:59
25	3	34	10.1	6'9"	7.1	161	2:01
20	3	31	10.2	6'7"	7.1	156	2:05
15	2	29	10.4	6'5"	7.2	150	2:09
10	1	26	10.6	6'2"	7.5	140	2:15
5	0	22	11.1	5'10"	7.7	125	2:25
0	0	0	13.9	4'2"	9.1	55	3:43

Motor Ability

Motor ability, the capacity to perform a variety of athletic events, has been thought to be a general indication of athletic ability involving balance, flexibility, power, velocity, timing, coordination, strength, endurance, agility, and the ability to learn a motor skill quickly. Among other things motor ability is affected by size, vision, rhythm, and previous experience with motor skills. However, research now indicates that such a general quality does not in fact exist; rather motor ability is specific to the task. Motor ability tests may however give an indication of past achievement in the factors measured. Since many of the components of motor ability are also those of physical fitness it would be expected that a relationship exists between the two; however, motor ability testing does involve some additional factors.

Most motor ability tests have been designed specifically for boys or girls, so we will present one test for each, although Scott's three-item test, originally designed for women, has been used with 9th grade boys and it would not be difficult to establish school or local norms for boys of other grades.

THREE ITEM TEST OF MOTOR ABILITY*

1. Obstacle Race

The space needed is 55 feet by 12 feet; equipment needed, three jump standards and a cross bar at least 6 feet long; lines on the floor (see Figure 2.14).

Description

Start in a back-lying position on the floor with the heels at line *a*. On the signal, *Ready, Go!* get up and start running toward J. As you come to each square on the floor, step on it with both feet. Run twice around J, turn back to d, go under the cross bar, get up on the other side, run to line *c* and continue running between line *b* and *c* until you come to *c* for the third time. The score is the number of seconds (to the nearest .1 second) that is required to run the course.

Suggestions

Give instructions to all the class so repetition is not necessary when individuals are ready to run. Demonstrate what is meant by stepping with both feet on each square.

---

*Scott, M. Gladys, and Esther French, *Measurement and Evaluation in Physical Education*, Dubuque, Iowa: Wm. C. Brown Company Publishers, 1959. Used by permission of the publishers.

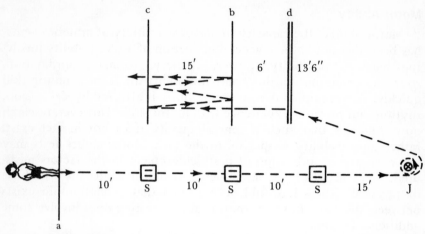

a	=	starting line.
b	=	line for shuttle.
c	=	finish line.
d	=	cross-bar (18 inches high).
J	=	jump standard
S	=	spot on floor (12 x 18 inches).
- - - -	=	path of runner

Distance from end of cross-bar to line of inner sides of spots, 4 feet 4 inches.

Figure 2.14. Floor Markings for Obstacle Race.

Each successive runner should lie down as soon as the girl ahead is up. This avoids delay in starting new runners.

If two timers and watches are available, the next girl starts as soon as the one ahead finishes circling the standard. Approximately twice the number can be scored on the same course with this arrangement.

Do not call the runner back if the toe or heel extends outside of the square. Some feet are too large to fit inside the square if the heel is lowered. Judge performance on whether the stride is adjusted to contact the square and whether there is a transfer of weight from one foot to the other while in the square.

2. Basketball Throw for Distance

Space needed is about 80 feet long and 20 feet wide, a throwing line marked about 8 feet from one end of the course and parallel lines every 5 feet beginning 15 feet in front of the throwing line.

Description

Start anywhere you wish behind the throwing line, but do not step on or across the line when throwing. Throw in any way you wish, three consecutive times. The score is the distance from the throwing line to the spot where the ball touches the floor. Only the longest throw counts.

Suggestions

Explain carefully but do not demonstrate. Answer questions about the test, except those on throwing technique. If asked whether the throw should be overhand or underhand, whether from a stationary position or with a step or run, simply reply that the throw may be of any type providing the feet are kept behind the line; the purpose is to throw the ball as far as possible. This may not be good teaching procedure, but it is essential for this form of testing if you wish to know how the student is likely to meet similar problems of throwing in a game.

It is true that some will profit more than others from seeing other students perform, but they are also the ones who learn quickly from class instruction. The ones who do not profit from errors or success of classmates doubtless will be slow to profit from class instruction.

If the gymnasium is too short and the test cannot be given outside, a diagonal course across the gymnasium may be used. This insures sufficient distance in practically any gymnasium but leaves little space in which to carry on other class activities during the test.

3. Standing Broad Jump

If the test is given outside, it is necessary to have a jumping pit with sunken take-off board within 30 inches of the edge of the pit. If given indoors, the test requires mats at least 7 1/2 feet long and a solid board at least 2 feet long (beat boards used with apparatus are excellent) placed against the wall to prevent slipping. If the mat is marked in 2-inch intervals, it eliminates the need to measure each jump with a tape.

Description

Stand on the take-off board with feet parallel, toes may be curled over the edge of the board. Take-off from both feet simultaneously; jump as far forward as possible. The score is the distance from the edge of the take-off board to the nearest heel (or to the nearest part of the body if the balance is lost). The best of three trials will be counted.

Suggestions

Preliminary swinging of arms and flexing of knees are permissible providing the feet are kept in place on the board until the actual take-off.

Be sure the performer understands what is to be done. The two-footed take-off is the point most frequently not comprehended from the description.

When the use of a take-off board is not feasible, jumping may be done from the mat if the mat is heavy enough that it will not slip.

Table 2.18.
Scott Motor Ability Test
Three Item
(Senior High)

T-Score	Basketball Throw (Ft.)	Broad Jump (In.)	Obstacle Race (Sec.)	Senior High G.M.A.
80	71			
79		96		
78				226
77	68	94		
76	66		18.5-18.9	
75	65			
74	64	92		
73	63			
72	61			222
71	59	90		218
70	55	88	19.0-19.4	214
69	54			208
68	52	86		204
67	51		19.5-19.9	198
66	50			194
65	49			192
64	48	84	20.0-20.4	190
63	47			188
62	46	82	20.5-20.9	182
61		80		178
60	45			172
59	44	78	21.0-21.4	170
58	43			168
57	42	76	21.5-21.9	166
56	41			164
55	40	74		162
54			22.0-22.4	160
53	39			158
52		72		154
51	37		22.5-22.9	150
50	36			148

T-Score	Basketball Throw	Broad Jump	Obstacle Race	Senior High
49	35	70		144
48		68	23.0-23.4	142
47	34	66		138
46	33		23.5-23.9	136
45	32	64		134
44	31		24.0-24.4	132
43		62		128
42	30		24.5-24.9	126
41	29	60		124
40	28			120
39		58	25.0-25.4	118
38	27	56		116
37		54	25.5-25.9	114
36	26		26.0-26.4	110
35		52	26.5-26.9	108
34	25	50	27.0-27.4	106
33				102
32	24	47	27.5-27.9	
31	23			100
30		44	28.0-28.4	96
29	22		28.5-28.9	92
28			29.0-29.4	90
27	21		29.5-29.9	
26		40	30.0-30.4	88
25	20			84
24			30.5-31.4	
23	19	36	31.5-32.4	78
22			32.5-34.9	
21	16			
20			35.0-36.0	

Table 2.19.
Scott Motor Ability Test
Three Item
(College Women)

T-Score	Basketball Throw (Ft.)	Broad Jump (In.)	Obstacle Race (Sec.)	College Women G.M.A.
85	75	86	17.5-17.9	234-235
84				
83	71		18.0-18.4	232-233
82				230-231
81		85		226-229
80	70			222-225
79	69		18.5-18.9	220-221
78	68	84		
77	67	83		218-219
76	66			214-217
75	65	82	19.0-19.4	212-213
74	64	81		210-211
73	62	80		208-209
72	61	79	19.5-19.9	204-207
71	59			200-203
70	58	78	20.0-20.4	194-199
69	57	77		192-193
68	56	76		188-191
67	55	75	20.5-20.9	186-187
66	54	74		182-185
65	52			178-181
64	51	73	21.0-21.4	176-177
63	50	72		172-175
62	48	71	21.5-21.9	168-171
61	47	71		164-167
60	46	70		162-163
59	45	69	22.0-22.4	158-161
58	44	68		156-157
57	43	67	22.5-22.9	152-155
56	42			150-151
55	41	66	23.0-23.4	146-149
54	40	65		144-145
53	39	64	23.5-23.9	142-143
52	38	63		138-141
51	37		24.0-24.4	136-137
50	36	62		132-135
49	35	61	24.5-24.9	130-131
48		60		128-129
47	34	59	25.0-25.5	126-127
46	33	58		122-125

T-Score	Basketball Throw (Ft.)	Broad Jump (In.)	Obstacle Race (Sec.)	College Women G.M.A.
45	32	57	25.5-25.9	120-121
44	31			118-119
43		56	26.0-26.5	116-117
42	30	55		114-115
41		54	26.5-26.9	110-113
40	29	53	27.0-27.4	108-109
39	28	52	27.0-27.4	106-107
38			27.5-27.9	104-105
37	27	51	28.0-28.4	102-103
36	26	50		100-101
35		49	28.5-28.9	98-99
34	25	48	29.0-29.4	94-97
33		47	29.5-29.9	90-93
32		46	30.0-30.4	88-89
31		45	30.5-30.9	86-87
30	24	44	31.0-31.4	84-85
29		43	31.5-31.9	80-83
28	23	42	32.0-32.4	
27	21	41	32.5-32.9	78-79
26		40	33.0-33.4	76-77
25	20	39	33.5-55.9	74-75
24		38	34.0-34.4	72-73
23		37	34.5-34.9	68-71
22		36	34.5-34.9	66-67
21	19		35.0-35.4	64-65
20				60-63
19		35	35.5-35.9	
18				38-59
17	18			
16				
15				
14			43.5-43.9	
13		30	45.5-45.9	34-37

BARROW MOTOR ABILITY TEST*

Floor Plan and Space Requirement

If only one station of each test is employed, a single gymnasium provides ample space. Figure 2.15 shows the floor plan.

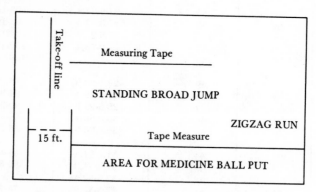

Figure 2.15. Floor Plan for Barrow Motor Ability Test.

Test Description

ITEM NUMBER I—STANDING BROAD JUMP (Figure 2.16A)

Purpose: To measure power primarily, and agility, speed, and strength secondarily.

Facilities and Equipment: One 5 by 12-foot tumbling mat marked with a take-off line and parallel lines two inches apart indicating distance from the take-off line. If the mat is not available, the floor can be used with a take-off mark and a tape measure.

Directions: The subject assumes the starting position behind the take-off mark with his feet parallel. He takes a preliminary movement by bending his knees and swinging his arms and jumps outward as far as possible. Three trials are permitted in succession.

Instructions: You should crouch before you jump and swing your arms downward. As you jump outward, the arms should be swung

---

*Barrow, Harold M., and Rosemary McGee, *A Practical Approach to Measurement in Physical Education,* Philadelphia: Lea & Febiger, 1964. Used by permission of the authors and publishers.

forward and upward. Take off from the mark with both feet simultaneously and try not to fall backwards after landing.

Scoring: The final score is the distance of the best jump measured to the nearest inch.

Testing Personnel: One trained assistant to supervise the testing station and measure and record the score.

ITEM NUMBER II—ZIGZAG RUN (Figure 2.16B)

Purpose: To measure agility primarily and speed secondarily.

Facilities and Equipment: Stop watch, five standards which are commonly used for high jumping, volleyball, or badminton. (If these are not available, chairs may be used.) Space for the zigzag course placed on the gymnasium floor with the standards placed at the indicated spots.

Directions: The event should be explained and demonstrated. The subject begins at the start and follows the prescribed course for three complete laps. The watch is stopped when the subject finishes his run at the end of the third lap.

Instructions: For the start of your run you may use a standing start. On the command to go you run the prescribed course in a figure-of-eight fashion. Do not grasp the standards as you round them and do not misplace them in any way. You complete three circuits of the course and continue to run past the finish mark. If you foul or fail to run the prescribed course, you will be required to run again.

Score: The final score is the elapsed time to the nearest tenth of a second which is required to run the prescribed course three times.

Testing Personnel: One trained assistant to supervise the testing station and to time and record the scores.

ITEM NUMBER III—SIX POUND
MEDICINE BALL PUT (Figure 2.16C).

Purpose: To measure arm and shoulder girdle strength primarily, and power, agility, arm and shoulder girdle coordination, speed, and balance secondarily.

Facilities and Equipment: A space in a gymnasium with approximately 90 by 25 feet. A restraining line is clearly marked with a second line 15 feet to the rear. The throw must be made from between these lines. The event may be measured with a tape measure but it will facilitate administration if concentric circles are placed.

Directions: The event must be explained and demonstrated since the try must be a put and not a throw. The subject stands between the two restraining lines and puts the ball straight down the course. He takes three trials in succession. Fouls count as a trial but in the event that all three trials are fouls, the subject must put until he makes a fair put.

Instructions: You must take up a position in the throwing area with the side opposite the throwing arm toward the line of the throw. You must put the ball and not throw it. You must not step on or over the restraining line during the throw.

Scoring: The final score is the distance of the best put measured to the nearest foot.

Testing Personnel: One trained assistant to supervise the testing station and to measure the throws and record the scores. Student assistants are needed to mark the spot of the throws and to return the balls to the throwing area.

Norms

Table 2.20. T-Scores For College Men

T-Score	Standing Broad Jump (Inches)	Zigzag Run (Seconds)	Medicine Ball Put (Feet)	T-Score
80	113 Up	20.8 Up	58 Up	80
75	109-112	21.6-20.9	55-57	75
70	105-108	22.4-21.7	52-54	70
65	101-104	23.2-22.5	48-51	65
60	97-100	23.9-23.3	45-47	60
55	93-96	24.7-24.0	42-44	55
50	89-92	25.5-24.8	39-41	50
45	85-88	26.3-25.6	35-38	45
40	81-84	27.1-26.4	32-34	40
35	77-80	27.8-27.2	29-31	35
30	73-76	28.6-27.9	26-28	30
25	69-72	29.4-28.7	23-25	25
20	68 Down	29.5 Down	22 Down	20

Table 2.21. Junior High School Boys

Grade	7	8	9	10	11	
T-Score						T-Score
80	9C Up	97 Up	103 Up	105 Up	112 Up	80
75	86-89	92-96	98-102	101-104	107-111	75
70	82-85	88-91	93-97	97-100	103-106	70
65	77-81	83-87	88-92	92-96	97-102	65
60	73-76	78-82	83-87	88-91	93-96	60
55	69-72	73-77	79-82	83-87	88-92	55
50	65-68	69-72	74-78	79-82	83-87	50
45	61-64	64-68	69-73	75-78	78-82	45
40	56-60	59-63	64-68	71-74	74-77	40
35	52-55	54-58	59-63	66-70	69-73	35
30	48-51	50-53	54-58	62-65	64-68	30
25	44-47	45-49	49-53	58-61	59-63	25
20	43 Down	44 Down	44 Down	57 Down	58 Down	20

Table 2.22. Zigzag Run T-Scores for High School and Junior High School Boys

Grade	7	8	9	10	11	
T-Score						T-Score
80	20.1 Down	17.8 Down	20.2 Down	21.6 Down	21.5 Down	80
75	21.4-20.2	19.5-17.9	21.3-20.3	22.7-21.7	22.6-21.6	75
70	22.7-21.5	21.2-19.6	22.4-21.4	23.8-22.8	23.7-22.7	70
65	24.0-22.8	22.8-21.3	23.5-22.5	24.8-23.9	24.7-23.8	65
60	25.2-24.1	24.5-22.9	24.6-23.6	25.8-24.9	25.8-24.8	60
55	26.5-25.3	26.2-24.6	25.7-24.7	26.9-25.9	26.8-25.9	55
50	27.8-26.6	27.8-26.3	26.8-25.8	27.9-27.0	27.8-26.9	50
45	29.0-27.9	29.5-27.9	27.9-26.9	28.9-28.0	28.9-27.9	45
40	30.3-29.1	31.2-29.6	29.0-28.0	29.9-29.0	29.9-29.0	40
35	31.6-30.4	32.8-31.3	30.1-29.1	31.0-30.0	31.0-30.0	35
30	32.8-31.7	34.5-32.9	31.2-30.2	32.1-31.1	32.0-31.1	30
25	34.1-32.9	36.2-34.6	32.3-31.3	33.1-32.2	33.0-32.1	25
20	34.2 Up	36.3 Up	32.4 Up	33.2 Up	33.1 Up	20

Table 2.23. Medicine Ball Put T-Scores for High School and Junior High School Boys

Grade	7	8	9	10	11	
T-Score						T-Score
50	43 Up	45 Up	49 Up	50 Up	54 Up	80
75	38-42	43-44	46-48	47-49	51-53	75
70	35-37	40-42	44-45	44-46	48-50	70
65	33-34	37-39	41-43	42-43	46-47	65
60	30-32	34-36	38-40	39-41	43-45	60
55	27-29	31-33	35-37	37-38	40-42	55
50	25-26	28-30	32-34	34-36	37-39	50
45	22-24	25-27	29-31	32-33	34-36	45
40	19-21	23-24	27-28	29-31	31-33	40
35	17-18	20-22	24-26	27-28	28-30	35
30	14-16	17-19	21-23	24-26	25-27	30
25	12-13	14-16	18-20	22-23	22-24	25
20	11 Down	13 Down	17 Down	21 Down	21 Down	20

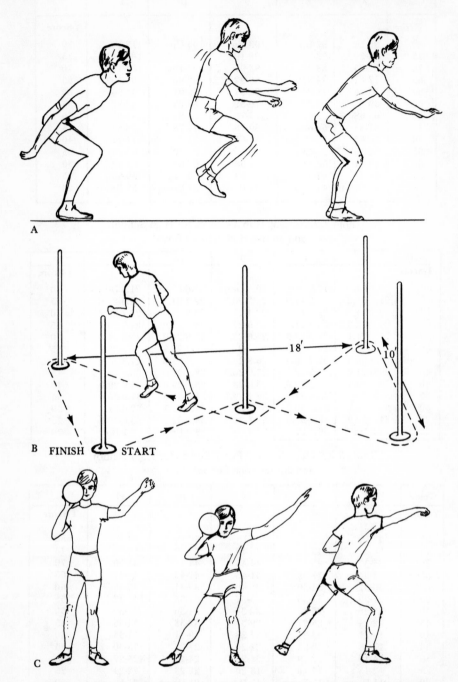

Figure 2.16. Test Items for the Barrow Motor Ability Test. A, Standing Broad Jump. B, Zigzag Run. C, Medicine Ball Put.

Posture

Posture is considered to be an indication of physical condition, Obviously muscular strength is involved in correct posture, and emotional condition is frequently reflected in carriage; some studies also tend to indicate a relationship between posture and ability to perform motor skills.[6] Many schools conduct posture programs and some school districts promote posture contests. A posture unit could be an addition to the program, but its inclusion necessitates being able to evaluate posture. This is somewhat difficult since the teacher must make all of the evaluations himself, or at least they must be made by a qualified observer.

Since many posture evaluation techniques involve difficult marking or special equipment, any method which will objectify what must be subjective judgments is helpful. Such a method is found in the posture test included in the New York State Physical Fitness test. Profile pictures are provided the rater for comparison with the student being rated, and a numerical score can be obtained from the test.

POSTURE TEST*

Posture is measured by reference to the rating guides for the 13 different segments identified on the Posture Rating Chart in the Cumulative Record Form. Each pupil must be rated individually by a qualified examiner.

a. Equipment and Testing Station

1. Heavy, clearly visible plumb line
2. Convenient stationary support for plumb line; e.g., horizontal bar
3. Masking tape (approximately 1 inch wide)
4. Backdrop or screen

Suspend a plumb line from a stationary support in front of an appropriate screen so that the bob almost touches the floor. Directly under the bob, construct a straight line using the masking tape. This line should begin at a point on the floor 3 feet from the bob toward the screen, pass directly under the bob, and extend 10 feet on the examiner's side of the bob.

---

*State of New York, *The New York State Physical Fitness Test: A Manual For Teachers of Physical Education,* Albany, N.Y.: Division of Health, Physical Education, and Recreation, New York State Education Department, 1958. Adapted by permission The State Department of Education.

b. Testing Procedure and Scoring

The pupil being examined assumes first a *comfortable and natural* standing position between the plumb line and the screen, straddling the short end of the floor line with his back to the plumb line. The examiner takes a position on the floor line about 10 feet from the pupil with the plumb line between himself and the pupil (Figures 2.17A and 2.17B).

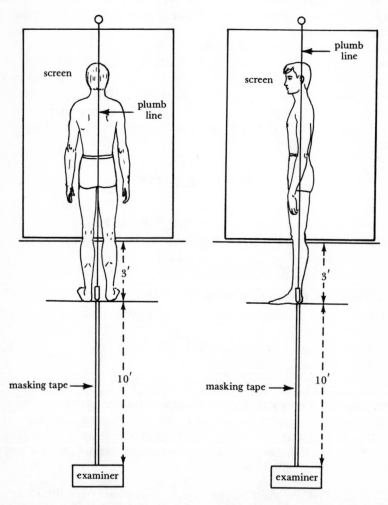

Figure 2.17 A. Position for Rating Lateral Posture.

Figure 2.17 B. Position for Rating Anteroposterior Posture.

After the pupil's lateral posture and feet have been rated, the pupil then makes a one-quarter left turn so that his left side is next to the plumb line, and stands with his feet at right angles to the floor line. His left ankle bone must be in line with the plumb bob (Figure 2.17 B).

Posture Rating Chart

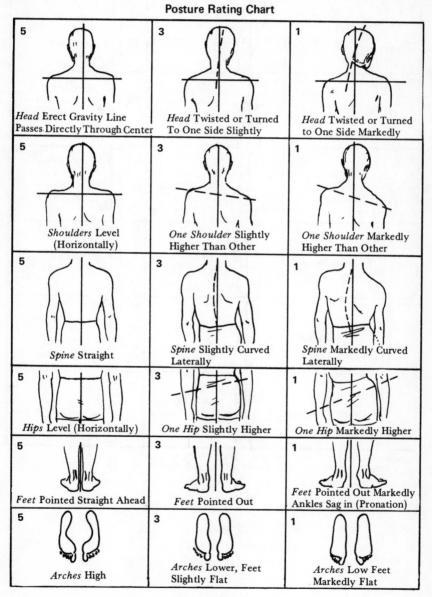

5	3	1
Head Erect Gravity Line Passes Directly Through Center	*Head* Twisted or Turned To One Side Slightly	*Head* Twisted or Turned to One Side Markedly
Shoulders Level (Horizontally)	*One Shoulder* Slightly Higher Than Other	*One Shoulder* Markedly Higher Than Other
Spine Straight	*Spine* Slightly Curved Laterally	*Spine* Markedly Curved Laterally
Hips Level (Horizontally)	*One Hip* Slightly Higher	*One Hip* Markedly Higher
Feet Pointed Straight Ahead	*Feet* Pointed Out	*Feet* Pointed Out Markedly Ankles Sag in (Pronation)
Arches High	*Arches* Lower, Feet Slightly Flat	*Arches* Low Feet Markedly Flat

Figure 2.17 C.

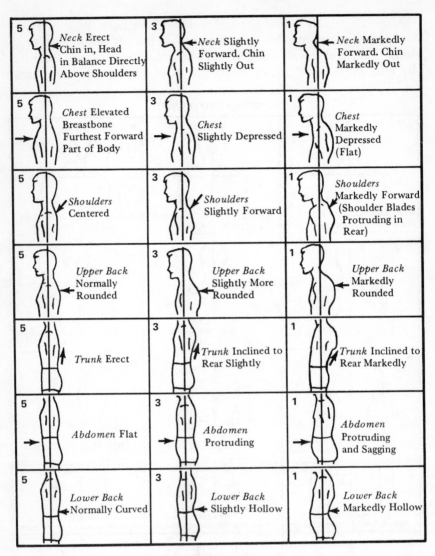

Figure 2.17 C. (con't.)

As the examiner scores each segment as shown on the Posture Rating Chart, he should first observe the pupil, then review the illustrations and descriptions on the rating chart, and, finally, evaluate the pupil and record his score in the box under the appropriate grade column. The pupil's score on each segment must be 5, 3, or 1. Each segment should be scored separately and the scoring of the previous segments should not be allowed to influence the score of the segment under consideration at the moment. The examiner should not be reluctant to enter extreme scores of ideal or markedly defective posture if they are merited. After ratings have been made for each of the 13 segments, record the total score in the space provided at the bottom of each page in the appropriate grade column. The sum of the 13 scores should, of course, be an odd number.

Another screening method, presented below, uses a posture evaluation sheet with stick figures representing lateral and posterior views. Symbols are placed on the diagrams to represent the various postural deviations. The instructor may devise his own symbols; however, some are suggested for your use.

EXAMPLE 1

NAME ————————

CLASS ————————

DATE ————————

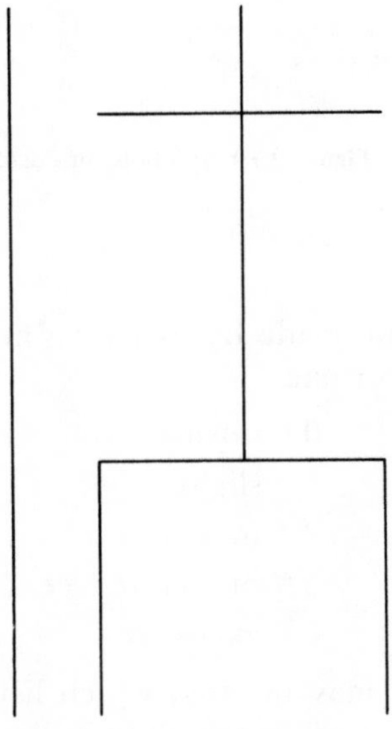

Figure 2.18. Posture Evaluation.

EXAMPLE 2

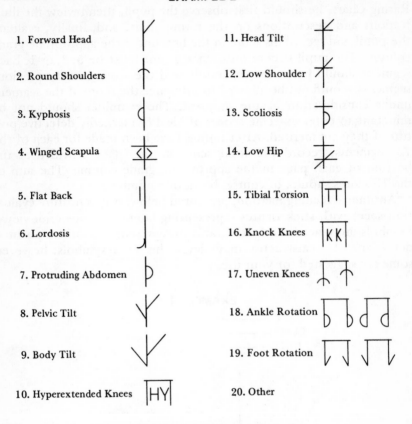

1. Forward Head

2. Round Shoulders

3. Kyphosis

4. Winged Scapula

5. Flat Back

6. Lordosis

7. Protruding Abdomen

8. Pelvic Tilt

9. Body Tilt

10. Hyperextended Knees

11. Head Tilt

12. Low Shoulder

13. Scoliosis

14. Low Hip

15. Tibial Torsion

16. Knock Knees

17. Uneven Knees

18. Ankle Rotation

19. Foot Rotation

20. Other

Figure 2.19. Symbols for Posture Evaluation.

Ratings may be made by assigning numerical values to degrees of deviation from normal.

> 0 = normal
> 1 = slight
> 2 = moderate
> 3 = moderate to excessive
> 4 = excessive

A rating scale may be used which lists the deviations; it is helpful to include also a space in which to indicate improvement.

EXAMPLE 3

POSTURE EVALUATION

Weight _____ ____

Height _____

Age _____

0 = Normal
1 = Slight
2 = Moderate
3 = Moderate to excessive
4 = Excessive

DEVIATIONS	IMPROVEMENT
1. Forward Head _____	_____
2. Round Shoulders _____	_____
3. Kyphosis _____	_____
4. Flat Back _____	_____
5. Lordosis _____	_____
6. Protruding Abdomen _____	_____
7. Pelvic Tilt _____	_____
8. Body Tilt _____	_____
9. Hyperextended Knees _____	_____
10. Head Tilt _____	_____
11. Low Shoulder _____	_____
12. Scoliosis _____	_____
13. Low Hip _____	_____
14. Tibial Torsion _____	_____
15. Knock Knees _____	_____
16. Uneven Knees _____	_____
17. Ankle Rotation _____	_____
18. Foot Rotation _____	_____
19. Other _____	_____

THE CONCOMITANTS

Objectives in physical education usually include several concomitants such as growth in social adjustment, sportsmanship, and the many factors which fall under the heading "attitude." Physical education can contribute to these things, but they present a monstrous task of evaluation. Since many of the concomitants are somewhat nebulous in definition and we are unable to state definitely what is involved, they are the most difficult to measure.

Most evaluation of the concomitants is done through the use of check lists, but there are some instruments which are valid to the extent that it is possible to define and measure the quality. Good validities in such cases are necessarily lower than those more easily measured.

Social Adjustment

There are two purposes which a measure of social adjustment can serve:

1. To identify the "fringers," those students who are not well accepted by their group, and

2. To evaluate growth in social adjustment as a result of the program.

Of course, changes in social status in the course of a year will not be entirely the result of the physical education class; but measures of friendship taken in the same group—physical education class—would certainly indicate changes within that group; some influences therefore might be attributed to the class. If the object is to identify the "fringers" the instrument would be administered at the beginning of the year and the classes structured to provide opportunities for those students to develop friendships and achieve acceptance. If the instrument is re-administered at the end of the term, changes in status would be indicated by the differences in scores.

The instructor may devise his own instrument, adapted to his situation, which would give him an indication of social acceptance. It is necessary only to describe a social situation and either have each student rated by every other student as on the next page, or have the students indicate their first, second, and third choices and score the student on the number of times he is chosen or rejected. An example of such a method is shown on page 54.

Cowell Personal Distance Ballot*

What To Do:	I Would Be Willing to Accept Him:						
	Into my family as a brother	As a very close "pal" or "chum"	As member of my "gang" or club	On my street as a "next door neighbor"	Into my class at school	Into my school	Into my city
If you had full power to treat each student on this list as you feel, just how would you consider him? How near would you like to have him to your family? Check each student in *one* column as to your feeling toward him. Circle your own name.	1	2	3	4	5	6	7
1.							
2.							
3.							
4. etc.							

Note: The Personal Distance Score is determined by adding the total *weighted* scores given the subject by members of the class or group and dividing by the total number of respondents. Division is carried to two places and the decimal point dropped. The low score is the desirable score. The percentile scale scores in the appendix represent boys' attitudes toward accepting boys. It is possible also to determing girls' attitudes toward girls, boys' attitudes toward girls and vice-versa by various methods of balloting.

*Cowell, Charles C., "Validating an Index of Social Adjustment for High School Use," *Research Quarterly*, 29, 7-18, March, 1958. Used by permission of the AAHPER.

EXAMPLE 4

Give first, second and third choices from this group for all items

---

1. With which class member would you most like to spend a free day?

    1.

    2.

    3.

2. With which would you *least* like to spend a day?

    1.

    2.

    3.

Scoring could be accomplished as follows:

EXAMPLE 5

Name	CHOSEN				REJECTED			
	1st	2nd	3rd	Total Times Chosen	1st	2nd	3rd	Total Times Chosen

This method will indicate *most* popular and *most* rejected by number of firsts in each category, and a general indication of acceptance and rejection through the "total times chosen" columns.

It might also be wished, for purposes of group construction, to use some method of identifying the respondent and, through sociometric tabulation, to find out who chose or rejected whom. (Obviously private information for instructor use only).

The value of such evaluation is to put together students choosing each other, or in the case of the "fringer," to place him with someone whom he has chosen who in turn has not rejected him, or who has chosen him.

Behavior

Behavior is usually measured by means of a rating scale scored by the teacher.

The instructor may design his own rating scale to include items not covered in the examples; he need only try to be careful to

SOCIOMETRIC TABULATION FORM*

Chosen ⟶ / Chooser	Ruth Allis	Irene Brown					Jos. Gold										John Smith		
Ruth Allis	•																		
Irene Brown		•																	
			•																
				•															
					•														
						•													
Jos. Gold	2	3					•									1			
								•											
									•										
										•									
											•								
												•							
													•						
														•					
															•				
John Smith																	•		
																		•	
																			•
Chosen as:																			
1st choice																1			
2nd choice	1																		
3rd choice		1																	
TOTAL																			

Sociometric Tabulation Form. List names in the same order vertically and horizontally. Insert a "1," "2," "3," in the proper squares to indicate the order of choices. Note example in the form: Joseph Gold chooses John Smith first, Ruth Allis second, and Irene Brown third.

*Helen H. Jennings, *Sociometry in Group Relations,* Washington, D.C.: American Council on Education, 1959, page 21. Used by permission of the publisher.

Behavior Rating Scale*

Name of Person Rated...　Grade.............Age.................

Name of Rater...　Date......................................

Rater's Assurance 0—a mere guess 1—slight inclination 2—fair assurance 3—positive assurance	Frequency of Observation							
	Rater's Assurance	No Opportunity To Observe	Never	Seldom	Fairly Often	Frequently	Extremely Often	Score
Leadership								
1. He is popular with classmates			1	2	3	4	5	
2. He seeks responsibility in the classroom			1	2	3	4	5	
3. He shows intellectual leadership in the classroom			1	2	3	4	5	
4. He lets others shove him around or take his place			5	4	3	2	1	
Positive Active Qualities								
5. He finds useful occupations when assigned tasks are finished			1	2	3	4	5	
6. He shows initiative in assuming responsibility in unfamiliar situations			1	2	3	4	5	
7. He exhibits aggressiveness in his relationships with others			1	2	3	4	5	
8. He is alert to new opportunities			1	2	3	4	5	
9. He quits on tasks requiring perseverance			5	4	3	2	1	
Positive Mental Qualities								
10. He shows keenness of mind			1	2	3	4	5	
11. He recovers his poise quickly after a failure			1	2	3	4	5	
12. He volunteers ideas			1	2	3	4	5	
13. He has the courage of his convictions; he does not conform when he disbelieves			1	2	3	4	5	
14. He teases and pesters others			5	4	3	2	1	
Self-Control								
15. He controls himself when provoked			1	2	3	4	5	
16. He is easily irritated			5	4	3	2	1	
17. He gets angry in arguments, discussions or debates			5	4	3	2	1	
18. He takes a justified criticism by teacher or classmate without showing anger or pouting			1	2	3	4	5	

*Blanchard, B.E. Jr., "A Behavior Frequency Rating Scale for the Measurement of Character and Personality in Physical Education Classroom Situations," *Research Quarterly*, 7, 56-66, May, 1936. Used by permission of the AAHPER.

Rater's Assurance 0—a mere guess 1—slight inclination 2—fair assurance 3—positive assurance	Rater's Assurance	No Opportunity To Observe	Never	Seldom	Fairly Often	Frequently	Extremely Often	Score
Cooperation								
19. He is willing to adjust to the interests of the group			1	2	3	4	5	
20. He is loyal to his group			1	2	3	4	5	
21. He discharges his group responsibilities well			1	2	3	4	5	
22. He is cooperative in his attitude towards the teacher			1	2	3	4	5	
23. He is willing to play without trying to run everything himself			1	2	3	4	5	
24. He grumbles over decisions of classmates or teachers			5	4	3	2	1	
Social Action Standards								
25. He is courteous			1	2	3	4	5	
26. He respects the rights of others			1	2	3	4	5	
27. He makes loud-mouthed criticisms and comments			5	4	3	2	1	
28. He shows off			5	4	3	2	1	
29. He is willing to admit ignorance or failure			1	2	3	4	5	
Ethical Social Qualities								
30. He tries to "get by" with bluffing			5	4	3	2	1	
31. He respects the rules			1	2	3	4	5	
32. He imposes on good nature			5	4	3	2	1	
33. He is truthful			1	2	3	4	5	
34. He cheats			5	4	3	2	1	
Qualities of Efficiency								
35. He is punctual at meetings, practice, classes			1	2	3	4	5	
36. He has good study habits			1	2	3	4	5	
37. He is dependable and trustworthy			1	2	3	4	5	
38. He finishes tasks he starts			1	2	3	4	5	
39. He plans things well			1	2	3	4	5	
40. He seems satisfied to "get by" with tasks assigned			5	4	3	2	1	
Sociability								
41. He is friendly			1	2	3	4	5	
42. He shows timidity			5	4	3	2	1	
43. He is liked by others			1	2	3	4	5	
44. He makes a friendly approach to others in the group			1	2	3	4	5	
45. He acts as though he felt abused or "picked on"			5	4	3	2	1	

Frequency of Observation (header spanning Never, Seldom, Fairly Often, Frequently, Extremely Often)

use statements of approximately equal distance or degree, especially if a total score is to be found for each student. If each item is to be considered separately, degree is not so important.

Social Evaluation Score Card*

Purpose

To provide the teacher with a guide for making a subjective appraisal of the social traits of his students.

General Procedures

A class roll can be used as the score sheet with a column designated for each trial. The students should not know when they are being rated.

Scoring

It is possible to make 50 points on the score card.

The Score Card

A. SPORTSMANSHIP
  5. Always displays good sportsmanship
  4. Most of the time is a good sport
  3. Has tendency toward poor sportsmanship
  2. Frequently displays poor sportsmanship
  1. Usually displays poor sportsmanship

B. ENTHUSIASM AND INTEREST
  5. Enters into all activities with enthusiasm and eagerness
  4. Has a few lapses in interest and enthusiasm
  3. When motivated is enthusiastic
  2. Is seldom enthusiastic
  1. Is rarely ever an enthusiastic performer

C. ATTITUDE TOWARD CLASS REGULATIONS AND MANAGEMENT
  5. At all times is a highly cooperative class member
  4. Cooperative most of the time
  3. Cooperative under duress
  2. Frequently uncooperative
  1. Uncooperative most of the time

D. EFFORT
  5. Always put forth best effort
  4. Put forth best effort most of the time
  3. Tries under motivation
  2. Frequently fails to put forth best effort
  1. Never tries

---

*Barrow, Harold M., and Rosemary McGee, *A Practical Approach to Measurement in Physical Education*, Philadelphia: Lea and Febiger, 1964. Used by permission of the authors and publishers.

E. SOCIABILITY
   5. Is always friendly and is well liked
   4. Is generally friendly and well liked
   3. Is frequently unsocial
   2. Is generally unsocial and not well liked
   1. Is withdrawn from the group

F. LANGUAGE
   5. Never uses profane or improper language
   4. Has one or two lapses
   3. Occasionally uses improper language
   2. Frequently uses profane language
   1. Daily uses improper language

G. RESPONSIBILITY AND DEPENDABILITY
   5. Never neglects duties and responsbilities
   4. Only occasionally neglects responsibilities
   3. Must be followed up frequently
   2. Frequently shirks responsibility
   1. Is completely undependable

H. APPEARANCE
   5. Is always in costume, neat and clean
   4. Only one or two violations of costume and hygiene regulations
   3. Occasionally violates regulations
   2. Frequently violates regulations
   1. Continually violates regulations

I. LEADERSHIP
   5. Uses initiative as a leader and is a good follower
   4. Can lead at times and is a good follower
   3. Is a good follower but has trouble leading
   2. Poor leader and is only a fair follower
   1. Never leads and is a poor follower

J. CARE OF EQUIPMENT AND SUPPLIES
   5. Uses good judgment and displays honesty
   4. Uses good judgment most of the time and is honest
   3. Frequently shows destructive tendencies but is honest
   2. Frequently shows destructive tendencies and lies out of it
   1. Is a destructive force in class

Attitude

Since one objective is continued participation in physical activities, it is considered important to determine students' attitudes toward physical education. Obviously, if a student does not enjoy or believe in the values of physical education, he will not continue participation; and this objective will not have been accomplished. Attitude is usually measured through a questionnaire or schedule in which the student indicates degree of agreement with a statement.

Physical Education Attitude Inventory*

Directions—Please Read Carefully: Below you will find some statements about physical education. We would like to know how you feel about each statement. You are asked to consider physical education *only* from the standpoint of its place as an activity course taught during a regular class period. No reference is intended in any statement to interscholastic or intramural athletics. People differ widely in the way they feel about each statement. There are no right or wrong answers.

You have been provided with a separate answer sheet for recording your reaction to each statement. (a) Read each statement carefully, (b) go to the answer sheet, and (c) opposite the number of the statement place an "x" in the square *which is under* the word (or words) which best expresses your feeling about the statement. After reading a statement you will know at once, in most cases, whether you *agree* or *disagree* with the statement. If you *agree,* then decide whether to place an "x" under "agree" or "strongly agree." If you *disagree,* then decide whether to place the "x" under "disagree" or "strongly disagree." In case you are undecided (or neutral) concerning your feeling about the statement, then place an "x" under "undecided." Try to avoid placing an "x" under "undecided" in very many instances.

Wherever possible, let your own personal experience determine your answer. Work rapidly, do not spend much time on any statement. This is not a test, but is simply a survey to determine how people feel about physical education. Your answers will in no way affect your grade in any course. In fact, we are not interested in connecting any person with any paper—so please answer each statement as you actually feel about it. *Be sure to answer every statement.*

Statements

1. If for any reason a few subjects have to be dropped from the school program physical education should be one of the subjects dropped.
2. Associations in physical education activities give people a better understanding of each other.
3. Physical education activities provide no opportunities for learning to control the emotions.

*Wear, Carlos L., "The Evaluation of Attitude Toward Physical Education as an Activity Course," *Research Quarterly,* 22, 114-126, March, 1951. Used by permission of the AAHPER.

4. Engaging in vigorous physical activity gets one interested in practicing good health habits.

5. Physical education is one of the more important subjects in helping to establish and maintain desirable social standards.

6. The time spent in getting ready for and engaging in a physical-education class could be more profitably spent in other ways.

7. Vigorous physical activity works off harmful emotional tensions.

8. A person's body usually has all the strength it needs without participation in physical education activities.

9. I would take physical education only if it were required.

10. Participation in physical education activities tends to make one a more socially desirable person.

11. Participation in physical education makes no contribution to the development of poise.

12. Physical education in schools does not receive the emphasis that it should.

13. Because physical skills loom large in importance in youth it is essential that a person be helped to acquire and improve such skills.

14. Physical education classes are poor in opportunities for worthwhile social experiences.

15. Calisthenics taken regularly are good for one's general health.

16. A person would be better off emotionally if he did not participate in physical education.

17. Skill in active games or sports is not necessary for leading the fullest kind of life.

18. It is possible to make physical education a valuable subject by proper selection of activities.

19. Physical education does more harm physically than it does good.

20. Developing a physical skill brings mental relaxation and relief.

21. Associating with others in some physical education activity is fun.

22. Physical education classes provide nothing which will be of value outside of the class.

23. Physical education classes provide situations for the formation of attitudes which will make one a better citizen.

24. There should not be over two one-hour periods per week devoted to physical education in schools.

25. Physical education situations are among the poorest for making friends.
26. Belonging to a group, for which opportunity is provided in team activities, is a desirable experience for a person.
27. There is not enough value coming from physical education to justify the time consumed.
28. Physical education is an important subject in helping a person gain and maintain all-round good health.
29. Physical education skills make worthwhile contributions to the enrichment of living.
30. No definite beneficial results come from participation in physical education activities.
31. People get all the physical exercise they need in just taking care of their daily work.
32. Engaging in group physical education activities is desirable for proper personality development.
33. All who are physically able will profit from an hour of physical education each day.
34. Physical education activities tend to upset a person emotionally.
35. Physical education makes a valuable contribution toward building up an adequate reserve of strength and endurance for every-day living.
36. For its contributions to mental and emotional well-being physical education should be included in the program of every school.
37. Physical education tears down sociability by encouraging people to attempt to surpass each other in many of the activities.
38. I would advise anyone who is physically able to take physical education.
39. Participation in physical education activities makes for a more wholesome oulook on life.
40. As far as improving physical health is concerned a physical educa-tion class is a waste of time.

Scoring

As previously explained there are five possible responses to each Inventory item: strongly agree, agree, undecided, disagree, and strongly disagree. The response considered most favorable to physical education receives a score of 5. Thus the above responses would be scored 5-4-3-2-1 or 1-2-3-4-5 depending on whether the item was worded positively or negatively. A subject's score on the Inventory is the sum of the scores made on the individual items. According to this method of scoring, a high score would indicate a favorable attitude toward physical education.

Table 4 gives normalized T-scores which were derived from the Short Form raw scores of the population of 472 college men.

Table 2.24.
T-Scores Corresponding to Given Raw Scores

R	T	R	T	R	T	R	T	R	T	R	T
200	78	175	60	150	47	125	38	100	31	75	26
199	77	174	59	149	47	124	38	99	31	74	25
198	76	173	59	148	46	123	37	98	30	73	25
197	75	172	58	147	46	122	37	97	30	72	25
196	74	171	58	146	46	121	37	96	30	71	25
195	73	170	57	145	45	120	36	95	30	70	25
194	72	169	56	144	45	119	36	94	30	69	25
193	72	168	56	143	44	118	36	93	29	68	24
192	71	167	56	142	44	117	36	92	29	67	24
191	70	166	55	141	43	116	35	91	29	66	24
190	69	165	54	140	43	115	35	90	29	65	24
189	68	164	54	139	43	114	35	89	28	64	24
188	68	163	53	138	42	113	34	88	28	63	24
187	67	162	53	137	42	112	34	87	28	62	23
186	66	161	52	136	42	111	34	86	28	61	23
185	66	160	52	135	41	110	34	85	28	60	23
184	65	159	51	134	41	109	33	84	27	59	23
183	64	158	51	133	41	108	33	83	27	58	23
182	64	157	50	132	40	107	33	82	27	57	23
181	63	156	50	131	40	106	33	81	27	56	23
180	63	155	50	130	40	105	32	80	27	55	22
179	62	154	49	129	39	104	32	79	26	54	22
178	62	153	49	128	39	103	32	78	26	53	22
177	61	152	48	127	39	102	32	77	26	52	22
176	60	151	48	126	38	101	31	76	26	51	22

Sportsmanship

Sportsmanship is a term frequently used, associated with sports, and about which there is some dissimilarity among definitions. We teach for sportsmanship and insist that it be exercised; and, therefore, it should be measured. This is perhaps the most difficult concomitant to measure, partly because of the gap between knowledge and action. The student may know the proper behavior, but pressures exist which make it difficult to act in a sportsmanlike manner in the heat of the game. Barrow's Social Evaluation score card includes sportsmanship as an item, and a student's score on this item reflects his actions. Haskins has developed a written test of sportsmanship which measures knowledge of, and attitudes about sportsmanship situations on the assumption that knowledge precedes attitude formation, which in turn precedes action. This test is designed as a teaching device, as well as a measure of sportsmanship knowledge.

ACTION-CHOICE TESTS FOR
COMPETITIVE SPORTS SITUATIONS*

Form A
•

A1. A football team's linesman gathers hands full of grass or dirt to throw into the opposing line's faces. This enables them to break through the opponent's line freeing their backs to make long runs and score touchdowns.

    a.   It is the official's fault for failing to penalize the players for such actions.

    b.   As long as the officials can't see the linesman do this they might as well try it.

    c.   The opponents should throw dirt or grass at this team when they get the chance in order to pay them back.

    d.   The other team has equal opportunity to try the same thing, therefore, this team is justified in its actions.

    e.   The linesmen's actions are unfair to the opponents and not in the spirit of the game.

A2. In little league baseball competition the coaches of some of the teams have been known to tell their players to participate in the "Stamp Act." The Stamp Act means that the players are to try to stamp on the umpire's feet whenever they can get close to him. The stamping is a means of protesting an umpire's decision. Whenever a disputed decision occurs the coach calls out "Stamp Act" and the players carry out the play.

    a.   Rather than argue, the players have an effective means of protesting the umpire's decision when they use the "Stamp Act."

    b.   The coach has no business telling his players to do such a thing.

    c.   The players should carry out the Stamp Act since the coach says this is a good maneuver.

    d.   This action is all right to use as long as the players do not really hurt the umpire by stamping on him.

    e.   This action is all right as long as the umpire knows why the players are doing the Stamp Act. It's all part of the game.

---

*By Mary Jane Haskins and Betty Grant Hartman. Copyright, 1960. Used by permission of the authors.

A3. Before face masks on football helmets were legalized by the rules, a team might wear them if the other team consented. Team A was playing team B. Team B's coach had consented to allow team A to wear masks. At half time the score was 21 to 0 in favor of Team A. Team B's coach protested the masks. Team B's coach heckled the officials all through the second half.

    a. Team B's coach had a right to protest since his team was losing.

    b. Team B's coach had no right to protest since he had already consented to team A wearing masks.

    c. The coach was correct in protesting but not heckling the officials during the second half.

    d. The officials should have allowed team B's protest and had team A remove the masks the second half.

    e. Team B should have put on masks to even their chances, rather than protest team A's wearing them.

A4. An outstanding All-American football player was known for his rough, tough play. When he started to tackle or block an opponent he never stopped even though the opponents might have handed the ball or they were obviously out of the play. When asked why he played this way he expressed the opinion that once he started for a player he could not stop. If he stopped suddenly he might injure himself.

    a. Little regard for opponents made him an outstanding player. Those who play football should expect such action from opponents.

    b. The All-American was right to avoid injury to himself.

    c. The All-American should be penalized for such roughness, especially when the person tackled or blocked was not involved in the play.

    d. To play roughly is bad enough, but to out and out admit it was because he was protecting himself, is even worse.

    e. This player is not a true All-American. Good players should consider their opponent's safety as well as personal safety. He should be able to stop.

A5. Two rival teams in a well-known conference played a basketball game on one of these team's home court. During this game, the visiting team's star player was consistently booed whenever he missed a basket, pass, rebound, or maneuver. In the return game on the other team's court, the home crowd took revenge by booing all the players on the opposition. They were retaliating for what the other team's home crowd had done to their star.

    a. Booing is a good device to use to rattle a player. If this could help the home team in the first game, such action is all right.

    b. "Getting back" at the other team during the return game was justifiable under the circumstances.

    c. Even though the star player had been booed the other team's crowd should not have paid them back.

    d. Booing individual players does more good than booing the whole team. In the second game, the spectators should have singled out one player.

e.   Players should learn to play under difficult situations. Having the crowd boo them helps them to ignore future experiences of the same nature.

A6.   A coach of a college football team taught the end player to use his knee on the head of the opposing backfield player. He was to use this whenever the opponent was trying to prevent the end tackling the kicker. After the end had used this maneuver several times the opposing blocker would become afraid of the end and let him by. The end player could never bring himself to follow his coach's instructions.

It is possible that player's knees can come in contact with an opponent's head during blocks, tackles, or evasive action; however, if this is done deliberately the player could be penalized.

a.   Such an action in football is unnecessary. The coach who advised, and the player who would execute such action were wrong.

b.   This action would be all right as long as the blocker is not injured.

c.   The end player was right not to follow his coach's instructions.

d.   The end player should follow his coach's instructions even though he felt the instructions were wrong.

e.   This is a perfectly good maneuver to use in football. The coach was right in advising it and the player wrong not to do it.

A7.   You are a member of a volleyball team and during a game your opponents hit the ball over the net. The ball barely grazes your fingers as it flys out-of-bounds. If you were this player what would you do?

a.   Tell the referee you touched the ball without waiting to see if anyone noticed your touching it.

b.   Wait to see if your teammates noticed your touching the ball. If they did not notice let the referee's decision stand.

c.   Since the referee did not notice your touching the ball and it is his job to make decisions, let his decision stand.

d.   Ask the opponents if they noticed whether you touched the ball. If they did not notice, do not report yourself to the referee.

e.   Since you discover that the opponents noticed that you touched the ball you should report yourself to the referee.

A8.   Second basemen, according to the rules of the game, must step on or tag second base before throwing to first base in making a double play. The runner who runs to second base from first base is put out in this manner and if the baseman's throw reaches first base before the batter arrives, the batter is out and thus a double play (or two outs) is made. Some big-league second basemen have been known to deliberately pretend to touch or tag second base, but miss. This allows them to cut down on the time it takes to touch second base and throw to first base, and enables them to get more double plays.

a.   Since it is the umpire's job to tell whether or not the second baseman touches the base before he throws, it is all right for the baseman to pretend to touch to cut down on his time if he can get away with it.

c.   This maneuver does not always help the baseman to get a double play so he might as well try it.

d.   This is all right for big league players to use, but school or minor league players should not use it.

e.   This is taking unfair advantage of the other team and therefore should not be done.

A9.   A baseball team that is losing a game, realizes that an opposing player was called safe at first on a trapped fly ball. The catcher of this team argues that the ball was not trapped but legally caught. The argument continues and the catcher calls the umpire names. The umpire finally evicts the catcher from the game.

a.   No player, regardless of the team he is on, should argue with an official.

b.   The catcher should not argue. He should expect the person who trapped the ball or some other teammate to do this.

c.   It would be all right for a player or catcher to argue as long as he feels the umpire is wrong and he is right.

d.   He was justified in arguing since his team was losing. If they had been ahead he did not need to argue.

e.   A player is justified in arguing with the umpire since this is customary in baseball, but he should not call him names.

A10.   A soccer player receives a chest high pass and taps the ball down to the ground with his hand. The referee does not see this foul. (Soccer players are allowed to play the ball with their feet, not their hands.) The soccer player goes on down the field with the ball.

a.   The player should raise his hand to indicate his foul to the referee.

b.   It is the referee's responsibility to see these fouls. If he fails to see them the player need not confess he fouled.

c.   The opponents should tell the referee the player fouled.

d.   As long as the player can get away with this action it is all right to use.

e.   This action may have been accidental. If the player does this again, the opponents should complain to the officials.

A11.   In a championship Little League Baseball game, the score was tied. In the final inning, with the last team at bat and a runner on third base, the following incident occurred: The third base coach, an adult, called to the rival team's pitcher and asked to see the ball. The young pitcher threw the ball to the coach, whereupon the coach stepped aside and let the ball go by. The runner on third base saw the ball rolling away and ran home scoring the winning run. There is nothing in the rules which states that such action is against the rules.

a.   The umpire should make the runner go back to third base even though he did not break a rule.

b.   The umpire should make the runner go back to third base, and speak to the adult about such tactics.

c.   The pitcher should have been smart enough not to do such a thing, therefore, what happened was all right.

d.   This is a perfectly good baseball maneuver and the adult coach was justified in using it.

e.   Such action is all right for older baseball players, but not for use on Little League players.

A12. Horse shows include events in which riders are judged on their ability and skill in riding. Other events involve judging the performance and appearance of the horse, not necessarily the skill of the rider, although a good rider can help a horse perform better. However, some horses perform well or poorly regardless of the skill of the rider.

During a horse show it became common knowledge that an outstanding horse, who was entered in an event where his performance was to be judged, was easily upset by loud whistles. A rival stable, wishing this horse to lose and their horse to win, stationed people around the outside of the ring. These people were to whistle loudly whenever the horse went by. The horse was upset, performed poorly, and lost the event. The rival stable's horse won.

a.   The whistling was unfair. The favored horse should be allowed to perform without distraction.

b.   The judge should have allowed the favorite to win since he must be aware of the distracting influences.

c.   The losing horse's owners should complain to the judges so they could stop the people whistling.

d.   Since the favored horse's weakness was common knowledge, the rival stable's action was justified.

e.   If the horse was really good and deserved to win, it should not be distracted by such actions and deserved to lose.

A13. Certain basketball teams are coached to set up plays which cause the opponents to foul. Some players and coaches believe this is clever basketball since the opponents may foul out of the game and their team may gain extra points by scoring on the free throws.

a.   Players should use such plays. The coaches are clever to direct their players in such fashion.

b.   Players who disagree with this type of play may learn them if their coach so directs but should not use such plays.

c.   Players should refuse to play for coaches who insist they use such plays.

d.   The players should tell their coaches they don't approve of such plays but use them if he insists.

e.   Officials, players, and coaches should agree not to use such plays.

A14. If a wrestler uses an illegal hold and hurts his opponent, the match is awarded to the victim. If an illegal hold is used and the opponent is not hurt, the opponent is awarded two points. During a wrestling match wrestler A used an illegal hold on wrestler B. The official awarded two points to wrestler B, but wrestler B's coach comes out and tells wrestler B he is hurt. Wrestler B insists he is all right but the coach says, "No—you are hurt." The referee had to award the match to the "hurt" wrestler B.

a. Since wrestler A used an illegal hold, wrestler B was right in pretending to be hurt and to take his coach's advice.

b. Wrestler B had no right to play "hurt" even though his coach told him to.

c. The referee should have been able to judge whether wrestler B was "hurt" or not. He should not have given the match to wrestler B.

d. The coach had no right to influence his wrestler B. His wrestler was put on-the-spot as was the official.

e. Wrestler A should not have used an illegal hold. Wrestler B's coach was right to tell his wrestler to be "hurt" to teach wrestler A a lesson.

A15. When a member of a swimming team entered a race he deliberately moved slowly into his position in hopes that it would upset his opponents and make them take false starts. His teammates, entered in other races, did the same thing. Swimmers are allowed to take their time in getting into position. If, however, the swimmers are obviously stalling, they could be penalized. This is difficult for officials to determine.

a. The opponents of these swimmers should learn not to be upset by such actions.

b. This is all right to try since it probably works only on poor swimmers.

c. This is all right since the opponents are not good enough to control their starting.

d. The opponents will eventually catch on and would actually profit by having this trick used against them.

e. These swimmers are taking unfair advantage of the opponents.

A16. A rather good golfer constantly tries to improve his opponent's game. He constantly offers advice on every shot, tells the opponent what club to use, and so forth.

a. The good golfer gives the appearance of knowing all there is to know. This is annoying to his opponent.

b. A good golfer should know that unasked-for advice may upset his opponents. He should refrain from this practice.

c. Such advice may be helpful to his opponents.

d. A good golfer should know that in tournament play a golfer may receive advice only from his caddy and therefore should not advise his opponents.

e. Since his intentions are to be helpful his actions shouldn't bother his opponents.

A17. In basketball the spectators and players often attempt to put pressure on the officials by booing, talking, and yelling. This is a way of pressuring the officials into becoming aware that the players and spectators expect them to give the close decisions to their team.

a. This is perfectly all right.

b. This is customarily done and is a good way of putting the officials "on their toes."

c. It is all right to yell and talk but not to boo.

d. The spectators should assume that the officials try to be fair, therefore, they should refrain from such action.

e. Such action probably does no good whatsoever so this is useless.

A18. During a football game an ineligible pass receiver catches a long touchdown pass and scores. The officials fail to determine that the player was ineligible. The score is allowed to stand.

a. The ineligible receiver should have confessed he was ineligible.

b. Since the officials did not see the error the player was justified in keeping his ineligibility secret.

c. The coach or teammates of the ineligible pass receiver should tell the officials about the error.

d. The players or coach of the opposing team should let the officials know they had made a mistake.

e. Since the officials did not see the error nothing should be done.

A19. The crowd booed their basketball coach when he removed a player from the game. The crowd showed the coach, by their actions, that they wanted the player back in the game. After the game, the coach announced to the papers that he was justified in removing the player from the game since it was for the player's own protection.

a. The crowd has a right to disagree with the coach.

b. The crowd should leave the decisions to the coach and refrain from criticizing.

c. The crowd has a right to disagree but should not boo.

d. The coach knows more about the game than the crowd so the crowd should realize this and stop their criticisms.

e. The crowd's action is not unusual, and is unimportant in its effect on players or coaches.

A20. In informal golf matches when there are no officials to watch each competing player, some players fail to count all the strokes they take. This gives them better scores and sometimes they end up winning the match.

a. The player who fails to count his strokes is actually harming his golf game. He never knows how well or how badly he is really playing.

b. Since this occurs in informal matches it doesn't matter whether players count their strokes or not.

c. This type of player may never be a good golfer nor win important matches. In important matches there are officials to check on players' scores and this practice would be uncovered.

d. Since there are no officials, players should be extra careful in scoring correctly and should call fouls against themselves.

e. This type of play is unfair and should not be tolerated.

Form B

•

B1. A football coach tells his boys how, when he played in college, he was told to stiff-arm the opposing star in order to put him out of the game. He laughingly tells of his success in achieving this assignment.

    a. To injure an opponent deliberately is wrong. By laughingly telling his players what he had done, the coach is setting a bad example.

    b. Putting opponents out of the game is clever. By telling them how he had achieved this, he showed his boys how they could do it.

    c. Since the coach had been taught to do this, he must think such actions are part of football, therefore, he was justified in setting such an example.

    d. Injuring players through legal means is good strategy. Any example in support of this belief should be used by the coach.

    e. Since his actions helped win the game the coach is justifiably proud of his achievement.

B2. A spectator at a basketball game sees that an opponent is about to shoot a free throw. He stamps, whistles, and tries to distract the player.

    a. If other spectators were trying to bother the player, you would also.

    b. Unless the officials stop you, you would try to bother the player.

    c. You would bother the player only if the score was close.

    d. You would not try to bother the player.

    e. If you were the only spectator trying to bother the player, you would stop.

B3. The timekeeper's whistle indicated the end of a wrestling match. The wrestlers continued even though the whistle had blown. During this overtime one of the wrestlers scored two points. The timekeeper informed the official that the two points had been scored after the match had been ended. The coach of the team that had scored the two points, argued with the official. The official compromised, since he was not sure when the match ended and the two points were scored in a legal maneuver. The official gave the scoring team one point and the match was tied.

    a. Since the two points were awarded the wrestler, the coach had a right to dispute with the official and gain a compromise.

    b. The coach should not dispute with the official since his wrestler's points were scored in an illegal overtime.

    c. The official had no right to compromise the situation. The two points scored were illegal and he should have accepted the timer's word.

    d. Since two points were scored as a result of the confusion over the timer's signal, the official was right to offer a compromise.

    e. The official should have allowed the two points to count since he wasn't sure they were not scored before the whistle.

B4.   At a particular field house where basketball games are played, the coach and substitutes for each team are seated underneath the basket, one team at one end of the floor and the other team at the other end.

Team A and team B are playing when suddenly the play comes down under team A's basket. Team A's coach stands up, leans over the shoulder of the official who is standing under the basket and points to a foul which he thinks the official should call.

a.   Team A's coach was correct in pointing out the foul to the official, only if the official missed the foul.

b.   Team A's coach should not have pointed out the foul because the official would probably call it anyhow.

c.   Team A's coach was wrong. He should let the officials do their job without interference, reminder, or attempts to influence their decisions.

d.   Team A's coach was doing his job as a good coach. His action serves as a reminder and keeps the officials alert.

e.   The coach's actions are justified since it is customarily part of his job to show the officials what they should call and what they are missing.

B5.   A tennis player is getting ready to play in a tennis match. While he is getting out his racket, putting on his tennis shoes, and warming up, he complains about not feeling too well. He continues, commenting that he knows he cannot play his best today. His comments seem to the spectators that he is trying to establish an alibi in case he should lose. He is defeated and after the match points out that he just wasn't playing his best today.

a.   Alibiing is a poor thing to do.

b.   If he genuinely felt bad, he has a right to mention the fact before or after the game.

c.   His remarks may be misunderstood by spectators as an alibi.

d.   Since such actions seem to the spectators like alibiing, the tennis player should not say such things.

e.   If the tennis player really felt bad he should not play. If he feels well enough to play he should keep still.

B6.   Football players are not allowed to move beyond the line of scrimmage until the ball has been snapped. Some coaches coach their teams and players to attempt to charge across the line of scrimmage a fraction of a second before the ball is snapped. This gives them an advantage over the defense since they outcharge them. The officials have difficulty in seeing this and the team may get away with this more times than they are caught.

a.   The coach and players are clever to be able to do this without being seen by the officials.

b.   If the officials can't tell whether the team is wrong, players have the right to try.

c.   Since the object of the game is to outcharge the opponents, any way they can do it is legal.

d.   This is against the rules so the players and coach are wrong to try to get away with such actions.

e. The opponents can do the same thing if they wish, therefore, teams are justified to try.

B7. During the last 30 seconds of a tied basketball game between two college teams, the players scrambled for a loose ball near team A's foul line. This resulted in a tie ball. After the official called the tie ball, team B requested time out and the official placed the ball on the foul line. After the time out, the official picked up the ball and awarded it to team A for a free throw, forgetting it was a tie ball. Team A's captain told the official he was wrong and the official accepted his word.

a. The official was correct in accepting team A's captain's word.

b. Team B should have corrected the official since they were being unfairly penalized.

c. The official should have continued with the free throw regardless of objections since he is in charge of the game.

d. Team A's captain should not have objected to the decision, he should have let team B's captain object.

e. Neither of the team's captains should attempt to change the official's decision. They should let the official discover his own mistakes.

B8. A previously undefeated tennis player was finally beaten in a close match. After the match and whenever someone spoke to him he would say, "I really didn't play my best game."

a. He had to say something when addressed. This was a good remark.

b. He was justified in making such a statement if he felt it to be true.

c. This was a clever remark. It should influence his opponent's opinion of him so that he might beat him later.

d. A good loser would never say such a thing.

e. Since this was the first time he had been beaten he was justified in making such a statement.

B9. In field hockey a player is permitted to hit the ball with her stick as hard as she wishes, as long as she does not hit the ball directly into an opponent. Sometimes a player hits when an opponent is very close. She hits the ball away and not at the opponent but in swinging the stick causes the opponent to duck or dodge to keep from being hit. This action is not illegal as long as the stick is not raised above the shoulders. Some players will not swing at the ball when an opponent is close but others concentrate on hitting the ball and expect the opponent to get out of the way of the stick.

a. Since there is no rule against this action, players are justified.

b. Players who swing at the ball when an opponent is standing close to the stick should be penalized.

c. If the players have not the nerve to play under such circumstances they should not participate.

d. Players should be coached to use and exercise caution in avoiding this type of play. It is better to lose the ball than to endanger an opponent.

e.   The object of the game is to get the ball. The first player to reach the
       ball has the right to do what she wishes.

B10. In league bowling one person will score approximately half the time, then a
     member of the opposite team scores the rest. This amounts to keeping
     score for about one and one half games. A bowler notices that the game
     being scored by the opponents is being scored incorrectly and in favor of
     the opponents.

a.   The bowler should call the matter to the attention of the opponents.

b.   The bowler should ignore the situation.

c.   The bowler should wait until his team is scoring and change the
       opponent's score.

d.   After the bowler calls the mistakes to the attention of the other team
       he should ask for a new scorer.

e.   If the error is pointed out and not corrected, the team should refuse
       to bowl.

B11. Player A is playing player B in a tennis match. Player A beats B in the first
     set, 6 games to 1. B continually stops to tie his shoes, wipe his face every
     few minutes, and moves slowly into position for each play. Player B dis-
     covers that these actions upset player A. He continues these maneuvers and
     beats player A in the second and third sets, winning the match.

a.   Player B is clever to use these tactics since they helped him win.

b.   Player A should use the same tactics against player B.

c.   Player B should not take unfair advantage of player A.

d.   Since player A could use the same tactics as player B, player B was
       right to use them.

e.   Player A, if he were a good player, would not let player B's tactics
       bother him.

B12. A basketball rule states that a captain of a team is the only player who may
     talk to an official, request time-out, or ask for permission to leave the
     court. Some players and coaches feel that if they constantly complain of
     being fouled when no foul occurred eventually they will gain an advantage
     by directing the attention of the officials to the opponents. It is possible
     this might work with some officials.

a.   Complaining about actual fouls is all right but not nonexistent fouls.

b.   This particular practice influences only a few officials, probably poor
       ones, therefore such action is all right.

c.   This is a good thing to do because it may help to determine which
       officials are good and which are not.

d.   This action is not in the spirit nor within the rules of the game and
       should not be practiced.

e.   Since this action is a violation of the rules, the officials should stop
       this practice and enforce the rule.

B13. A rider in a horse show is putting his horse through various maneuvers and
     "gaits" required in that particular event. For example, the rider rides the

horse through walk, trot, and canter with the judge estimating the skill with which the rider controls the horse and puts the horse through his paces. Another rider, in the same event, tries to crowd, shove, and annoy the first rider whenever the judge is not looking. If the judge sees the second rider doing these things, he can disqualify him, but unfortunately he does not. The first rider does not know what to do. He should:

a. Report the opposing rider's actions to the officials in charge of the show.

b. Ask the opposing rider to stop crowding and tell him that if he does not stop he will report him to the officials.

c. Ask the other rider to stop and threaten to crowd him if he does not stop.

d. Wait until the show is over and then report the opponent's actions to the show officials after telling the opponent he is going to do this.

e. Simply ignore the opposing rider and pretend that nothing is happening.

B14. A field hockey team is being badly beaten by their opponents. They finally get into position to score and as one player drives the ball toward the goal, her teammate inadvertently lets the ball bounce off her foot into the goal. The umpire does not see the kicking foul and indicates the goal is good.

a. The player who kicked the ball should tell the official what she did.

b. The teammates of the player who kicked the ball should tell the umpire.

c. The team which is ahead should inform the official that the goal was illegal.

d. Since the team scoring the goal was behind it is to their advantage to confess the foul so that the opponents will think more of them even though they are not playing too well.

e. The official's decision should stand.

B15. In a baseball game a base-runner was forced to run from first to second base when the batter hit the ball toward second. The base-runner was easily put out but he deliberately crashed into the second baseman who was trying to throw to first base, and who was not in the runner's way. It is common practice for runners to try to prevent basemen from throwing—by running into them. Although this is against the rules it is difficult for umpires to tell whether the runners are deliberately or accidentally knocking the baseman down.

a. Customary or not, the base-runner should have avoided the second baseman.

b. The base-runner runs the risk of being called out by the umpire, if he can get away with it, he might as well try.

c. The base-runner was doing what is common by running into the baseman in order to prevent another out.

d. The base-runner should get in the way of the second baseman rather than knock him down.

e. Basemen expect this type of action from base-runners, so it was a risk; he should expect such things to happen, and try to avoid the runner.

B16. In a World Series baseball game one of the pitchers had a no-hit, no-run game up to the last batter. In the last half of the last inning, the batter at bat had a count of 3 balls and 2 strikes. As the pitcher delivered the ball, the umpire called "Strike three, you are out." The batter objected violently but the game was over and the pitcher had won his no-hit, no-run game. Later, the batter told newspaper reporters that the third strike was wild and the umpire probably had called it a strike just to give the pitcher the glory of winning a no-hit World Series game. It was also known that the umpire in question was retiring and this was his last game.

a. Since winning a no-hit game in the World Series is almost unheard of, the umpire was justified in calling that last pitch a strike regardless of where the ball was. The batter's team would have lost anyway.

b. Big league umpires are very good and they very seldom make mistakes. The batter was wrong and the umpire was right.

c. The batter should not have protested the umpire's decision in the first place, much less go on to announce later that the call was wrong.

d. It was all right for the batter to object to the third strike during the game but he should not have said anything later.

e. It is possible the umpire was wrong but since he was retiring and the pitcher had done so well, he was justified in calling any kind of pitch "strike three."

B17. A field hockey player hit her opponent on the shins just as she was about to receive a pass from a teammate. The player who hit the opponent's shins intercepted the pass and went on to score. It is against the rules to hit a player with your stick but the official did not see the foul.

a. If the official did not see the foul the player need not confess she fouled.

b. The player should not have broken a rule. She should have indicated she fouled.

c. The opponent should wait for a chance to pay the player back and hit her on the shins.

d. Not all officials see all the fouls which may occur. Nothing need be done. If the player should foul again she will probably be caught.

e. If the teammates of this player realized she fouled they should tell the officials.

B18. The groundskeepers have sprinkled lime on home-plate to mark it more clearly. A runner slides into home-plate. The catcher, by sitting on home-plate, blocks the runner. The umpire calls the runner safe, but the catcher stands up and shows the umpire the imprint of home-plate on the seat of his pants. The catcher maintains the runner was out since he could not possibly touch home while he was sitting on home-plate. Blocking bases frequently occurs and is commonly accepted as good play although it is against the rules.

a. The catcher should object strenuously since he has unquestionable evidence that the runner could not have touched home-plate.

b. If the umpire does not change his decision, the catcher should appeal to the other umpire or officials.

c. You should accept the umpire's decision since he is the authority in the game.

d. You should accept the decision but argue anyhow to let the umpire know how you feel.

e. Blocking home-plate takes unfair advantage of his opponent. If he earned a run he should get it. The official's decision should stand.

B19. A fencer consistently makes comments, shouts, or stamps his feet as he attacks his opponent. This seems to upset his opponent, but the first fencer is not breaking the rules of the sport.

a. This is perfectly all right if the fencer is not breaking any rules.

b. If this is the only way this fencer can win, he is not really a good fencer, and should not do such a thing.

c. The coach or officials should advise the fencer to stop this action.

d. The opponent should tell the other fencer what he thinks of such action.

e. Shouting, stamping, etc., are not in the "spirit" of fencing. Fencers should not do these things.

B20. A baseball player trapped a fly ball between the ground and his glove in what appeared to be a spectacular catch. Such action is called "Trapping" and is against the rules. The player wasn't sure the umpire saw him.

a. The player should have immediately confessed that he illegally trapped the ball.

b. The player should wait for the umpire's decision and abide by it.

c. If the umpire ruled his catch illegal, he should disagree on the grounds that he felt that the umpire could not see the play.

d. If the umpire asks him if he trapped the ball he should say he did.

e. If the umpire asks him, he should say he did not trap the ball.

KEYS

Form A		Form B	
1. e	11. b	1. a	11. c
2. b	12. a	2. d	12. d
3. b	13. e	3. c	13. b
4. e	14. d	4. c	14. a
5. c	15. e	5. e	15. a
6. a	16. b	6. d	16. c
7. a	17. d	7. a	17. b
8. e	18. a	8. d	18. e
9. a	19. b	9. d	19. e
10. a	20. d	10. a	20. a

SPORTS SKILL TESTING

Achievement of skill in the activities taught comprises the major part of a testing program. Skills are the tools with which we work, through which we achieve most of our objectives, and upon which we should base the major part of our grade.

When selecting a skill test the instructor must consider:

1. Its ease of administration: time required, space, equipment, and personnel necessary.
2. Its scientific authenticity: is it valid and reliable?

Many skill tests have been published and may be found, with a little digging, in measurement texts, sports guides, and research reports.

Some activities do not lend themselves well to skill testing, and the reader is referred to the section on rating scales and check lists for their evaluation.

One or more skill tests in several activities are presented, and the bibliography refers the reader to other sources.

ARCHERY SKILLS TEST*

Purpose

To measure accuracy in shooting with a bow and arrow at a standard 48-inch archery target from Distance A—10 yards, Distance B—20 yards, and Distance C—30 yards.

Equipment

A shooting range on level ground of at least 200 feet in length and 50 feet in width for each archery target in use. Standard 48-inch face archery targets placed on suitable stands so that the center of the target is 48 inches above the ground.

When the test is given indoors a gymnasium floor at least 96 feet in length, with appropriate backstops behind the targets will be needed.

Bows of assorted strengths of pull from 15 to 40 pounds should be available depending upon the age and ability of archers being tested.

Arrows of 24 to 28 inches in length to fit the bows and archers, with 8 to 10 arrows of the same color for each archer. Archers may use their own equipment if it is inspected and safe.

---

*AAHPER, *Archery Skills Test Manual,* Washington, D.C. American Association for Health, Physical Education, and Recreation, (1201 16th Street, N.W., Washington, D.C.). Used by permission of the AAHPER.

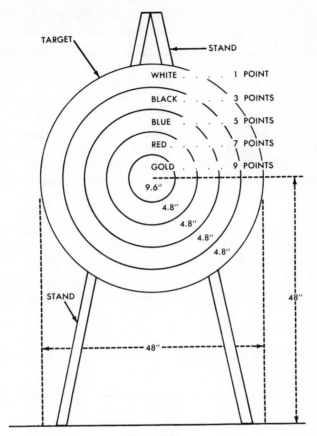

Figure 2.20.

Each archer should have arm guard, finger tab or glove, and quiver.

Other equipment includes line marker, stakes, measuring tape, whistle, squad score cards, pencils, and class composite record sheet.

Description

The standard archery target is made of straw, and is usually mounted on a wooden tripod. The target face may be of oil cloth or heavy paper with five concentric circles, the center being 9.6 inches in diameter and the others 4.8 inches wide. The center circle is painted gold, followed by red, blue, black, and the outer circle white.

Squads of four archers only shoot at any one target.

Each archer will shoot two ends at each distance for which he or she qualifies. Each archer will shoot one end and be scored on these, and will then wait his or her turn to shoot the remaining end.

The scorer will withdraw the arrows and announce the score of each arrow as it is withdrawn. The recorder will record the score of each arrow on the squad score card. After each archer has shot 12 arrows the total score at the distance will be recorded.

After all archers of a squad have completed shooting two ends at Distance A, the squad will move back to the second Distance B, take their practice shots, and again shoot two ends as before. After completing shooting at Distance B, the squad (boys only) moves to Distance C and, after practicing, shoots two ends in rotation as before.

Archers will stand astride the shooting line while shooting. Any method of aiming can be used, i.e., bow sight, point of aim, or instinctive shooting. The archer may adjust the aim during the practice shots or during testing, but no additional practice shots will be allowed for this purpose. Archers who fail to score ten points at any distance may not be allowed to shoot at the next distance at the tester's discretion.

Rules

1. The archer must stand astride the shooting line while shooting.
2. Four practice shots at each distance are allowed.
3. The archer may adjust the point of aim during practice shots or during testing, but no additional practice shots for this purpose will be allowed.
4. Each archer shoots one end at a time, and then waits his or her turn to shoot the other end.

Scoring

Arrows hitting in the center or gold circle count 9 points, arrows hitting in the next or red area count 7 points, arrows hitting in the blue area count 5 points, arrows hitting in the blue area count 5 points, arrows hitting in the black area count 3 points, and arrows hitting in the outer or white area count 1 point. Arrows striking in two colors count the value of the higher scoring area. Arrows striking the target but falling to the ground count 7 points regardless of where they strike. The maximum score at each distance is 108 points, and the maximum score at the first two distances (for girls) is 216 points, while the maximum score for all three distances (boys) is 324 points.

Table 2.25

10 YARDS — 12 ARROWS (BOYS)
Percentile Scores Based on Age / Test Scores in Points

Percentile	12-13	14	15	16	17-18	Percentile
			AGE			
100th	91	96	100	100	100	100th
95th	83	88	97	99	98	95th
90th	78	80	94	97	96	90th
85th	73	78	90	96	93	85th
80th	70	75	88	91	90	80th
75th	67	72	84	90	88	75th
70th	64	70	80	88	86	70th
65th	61	68	78	86	84	65th
60th	59	67	76	84	82	60th
55th	57	65	73	80	79	55th
50th	54	63	69	79	77	50th
45th	50	60	65	77	74	45th
40th	48	57	62	75	71	40th
35th	45	55	59	72	68	35th
30th	42	52	55	70	63	30th
25th	38	45	51	67	59	25th
20th	34	40	48	61	55	20th
15th	31	36	43	51	48	15th
10th	26	31	36	50	40	10th
5th	16	25	25	40	27	5th
0	0	0	0	0	0	0

10 YARDS — 12 ARROWS (GIRLS)
Percentile Scores Based on Age / Test Scores in Points

Percentile	12-13	14	15	16	17-18	Percentile
			AGE			
100th	85	89	96	100	100	100th
95th	69	74	82	87	87	95th
90th	60	68	75	80	80	90th
85th	50	63	70	73	73	85th
80th	46	58	66	67	69	80th
75th	41	54	63	64	66	75th
70th	38	50	60	60	62	70th
65th	35	48	56	56	58	65th
60th	34	46	53	53	55	60th
55th	32	43	51	49	52	55th
50th	30	41	49	46	48	50th
45th	27	38	46	43	46	45th
40th	24	35	43	41	42	40th
35th	22	33	40	38	40	35th
30th	19	30	37	33	38	30th
25th	16	28	34	31	35	25th
20th	14	25	31	29	31	20th
15th	12	22	27	25	28	15th
10th	10	19	21	21	24	10th
5th	6	12	13	16	19	5th
0	0	0	0	0	0	0

Table 2.26

20 YARDS — 12 ARROWS (BOYS)

Percentile Scores Based on Age / Test Scores in Points

Percentile	AGE					Percentile
	12-13	14	15	16	17-18	
100th	70	75	90	100	95	100th
95th	53	61	77	78	78	95th
90th	44	48	70	71	72	90th
85th	38	45	66	67	67	85th
80th	34	41	63	63	63	80th
75th	31	38	58	59	59	75th
70th	28	36	54	56	55	70th
65th	26	33	51	54	52	65th
60th	24	30	47	51	49	60th
55th	23	28	42	48	46	55th
50th	22	26	39	46	43	50th
45th	20	24	36	43	40	45th
40th	18	22	34	41	37	40th
35th	16	20	31	39	34	35th
30th	14	18	28	36	32	30th
25th	12	16	24	33	29	25th
20th	10	14	21	28	25	20th
15th	8	12	18	25	20	15th
10th	6	10	15	20	17	10th
5th	3	6	9	14	11	5th
0	0	0	0	0	0	0

20 YARDS — 12 ARROWS (GIRLS)

Percentile Scores Based on Age / Test Scores in Points

Percentile	AGE					Percentile
	12-13	14	15	16	17-18	
100th	60	70	81	91	95	100th
95th	40	47	55	58	71	95th
90th	29	38	47	50	60	90th
85th	22	35	43	44	52	85th
80th	19	32	39	40	47	80th
75th	17	28	34	36	42	75th
70th	15	25	32	32	40	70th
65th	13	23	29	29	36	65th
60th	12	21	27	27	32	60th
55th	10	20	25	25	29	55th
50th	9	18	23	22	26	50th
45th	7	16	22	20	24	45th
40th	6	14	20	18	21	40th
35th	1	12	18	16	19	35th
30th	0	10	16	14	18	30th
25th	0	8	13	12	16	25th
20th	0	7	11	10	14	20th
15th	0	0	8	8	12	15th
10th	0	0	6	6	9	10th
5th	0	0	0	0	0	5th
0	0	0	0	0	0	0

Table 2.27

30 YARDS — 12 ARROWS (BOYS)

Percentile Scores Based on Age / Test Scores in Points

Percentile	AGE					Percentile
	12-13	14	15	16	17-18	
100th	45	50	81	95	85	100th
95th	28	34	50	56	64	95th
90th	24	28	41	47	53	90th
85th	22	24	35	43	47	85th
80th	18	21	31	40	42	80th
75th	16	18	28	36	39	75th
70th	14	16	25	32	37	70th
65th	12	15	22	30	35	65th
60th	11	13	20	28	31	60th
55th	9	11	17	25	28	55th
50th	8	10	15	23	26	50th
45th	7	8	14	22	24	45th
40th	6	7	13	20	21	40th
35th	4	5	12	18	20	35th
30th	0	4	11	16	17	30th
25th	0	0	10	13	16	25th
20th	0	0	9	11	11	20th
15th	0	0	7	9	9	15th
10th	0	0	6	6	6	10th
5th	0	0	2	2	3	5th
0	0	0	0	0	0	0

Table 2.28

TOTAL OF 10, 20, AND 30 YARDS (BOYS)
Percentile Scores Based on Age / Test Scores in Points

Percentile	AGE					Percentile
	12-13	14	15	16	17-18	
100th	195	210	270	270	270	100th
95th	156	179	215	220	222	95th
90th	138	160	195	205	206	90th
85th	128	150	187	197	197	85th
80th	122	146	177	189	190	80th
75th	112	143	167	181	184	75th
70th	103	139	158	173	176	70th
65th	98	136	149	163	166	65th
60th	93	130	140	160	158	60th
55th	87	124	130	154	151	55th
50th	81	119	120	148	144	50th
45th	74	114	114	142	136	45th
40th	67	110	107	136	130	40th
35th	60	106	100	129	125	35th
30th	54	98	94	123	119	30th
25th	47	87	87	117	112	25th
20th	38	77	79	110	109	20th
15th	28	69	70	103	96	15th
10th	21	61	62	80	86	10th
5th	15	43	43	61	65	5th
0	0	0	0	0	0	0

TOTAL OF 10 AND 20 YARDS (GIRLS)
Percentile Scores Based on Age / Test Scores in Points

Percentile	AGE					Percentile
	12-13	14	15	16	17-18	
100th	129	159	160	161	180	100th
95th	100	109	130	134	149	95th
90th	89	99	112	115	129	90th
85th	81	89	103	107	123	85th
80th	69	84	96	100	116	80th
75th	64	79	89	96	109	75th
70th	60	75	85	91	104	70th
65th	55	70	80	87	100	65th
60th	50	66	77	80	95	60th
55th	46	62	73	76	91	55th
50th	42	58	70	72	85	50th
45th	38	54	66	67	78	45th
40th	35	50	62	63	73	40th
35th	32	47	59	60	68	35th
30th	28	45	55	56	64	30th
25th	25	42	51	52	60	25th
20th	22	40	45	47	53	20th
15th	17	34	40	41	45	15th
10th	12	28	33	36	38	10th
5th	5	22	25	26	30	5th
0	0	0	0	0	0	0

BADMINTON SKILL TESTS*
Short Serve (French)

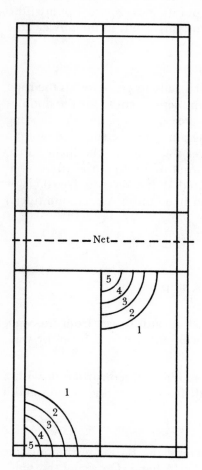

Figure 2.21. Floor Markings for Badminton Serve Test. 1-5 = Scores for Respective Areas, Right Court for Short Serve, Left Court for Long Serve.

Equipment

1. A clothesline rope stretched 20 inches directly above the net and parallel to it, attached to the same standards as the net. New shuttles and tightly strung rackets.

2. Floor markings.

Using the intersection of the short service line and the center line as a midpoint, describe a series of arcs in the right service court at distances of 22 inches, 30 inches, 38 inches, and 46 inches from the midpoint, the measurement including the width of the 2-inch line. Extend these arcs from the short service line to the center line, as indicated in the diagram (Figure 2.21). The lines should be painted in different colors to increase accuracy in scoring. Showcard paint, which be washed from the floor, is suggested.

Test

The player being tested stands any place in the right service area diagonally opposite the target, and serves twenty times, attempting to send the shuttle through the space between the rope and the net

---

*Scott, M. Gladys, and Esther French. *Measurement and Evaluation in Physical Education*, Dubuque, Iowa: Wm. C. Brown Co. Publishers, 1959, pages 144-158. Used by permission of the publishers.

in such a manner that it lands in the right service court for the doubles game. The scorer stands near the center of the left service court on the same side of the net with the target and facing the target. The corner of the target nearest the intersection of the short service line and center line counts 5 points, next space 4 points, the next 3, then 2, and any shuttle off the target but in the service area for the doubles games counts 1 point.

Scoring

No score is given for any trial which fails to go between the rope and the net or which fails to land in the service court for the doubles game. Any shuttle landing within an area or on the line surrounding an area is scored as shown in the diagram. Any shuttle landing on a line dividing two scoring areas receives the score of the higher area. The score for the entire test is the total of twenty trials. It is considered a foul and the trial is repeated if the serve is illegal. (For definition of legal serve, see American Badminton Association rules.)

Wall Volley No. 1 (Stalter)

Equipment

1. New shuttles, tightly strung rackets, stop watch.
2. Floor markings

Construct a restraining line parallel to and 6 feet from the wall, including the width of the line in the 6-foot distance from the wall.

3. Wall space

Use an unobstructed wall with smooth brick construction with a space of from 12 to 15 feet in width for each testing station and a height of at least 15 feet.

Test

The player to be tested stands behind the 6-foot restraining line facing the wall with racket and shuttle in hand. On signal, he sends the shuttle with an underhand serve against the wall and volleys it on each rebound for a period of thirty seconds. Strokes made while the player is touching the floor nearer the wall than the restraining line do not count. The player may cross the restraining line to recover the shuttle but he must return to behind the line before putting the shuttle into play again with an underhand motion. Any stroke may be used; hard driven forehands or backhands with good wrist action seem to produce the best results. The test should be demonstrated and a practice period should be allowed before any data are collected. (This wall practice can be used advantageously throughout the season by players waiting turns to get on the courts; if this has been done, the practice period on the testing day need not exceed one trial for each player.) The scorer stands behind the player and slightly to one side. The need for repeating trials due to foot faults can be minimized if the scorer immediately corrects the position of any player who steps on or over the restraining line. Twenty or more players can be tested at one time along the four walls of the usual sized gymnasium. Four trials are allowed for each player, recording all scores. The scorer and player to be tested should alternate to assure each of a rest period between trials.

Scoring

One point is scored for each volley against the wall. Putting the shuttle into motion with an underhand serve is not to be considered a volley. The score for the test is the total of the four trials.

Clear Test No. 1 (French)

Equipment

1. A clothesline rope stretched across the court 14 feet from the net and parallel to it, at a height of 8 feet from the floor.
2. Floor markings
   a. Construct a line 2 feet nearer the net than the rear service line in the doubles game and parallel to it. Measure from the exact center of the line. Extend this line from one outer alley line to the other outer alley line.
   b. On the same side of the net, construct a line 2 feet farther from the net than the rear service line in the singles game and parallel to it. Measure from the exact center of the line. Extend this line from one outer alley line to the other outer line. The lines should be painted different colors to increase accuracy in scoring.
   c. On the opposite side of the net, draw marks 2 inches square at spots indicated on the diagram as X and Y. The center of X should be 11 feet from the net and 3 feet from the center line toward the left side line. The center of Y should be 11 feet from the net and 3 feet from the center line toward the right side line. In measuring from the center line, use the exact center of the line.

Test

The player being tested stands between the two square marks on the court opposite the target. The person giving the tests (player with considerable experience) stands on the intersection of the short service line and the center line on the same side of the net as the target and serves the shuttle to the player being tested. The shuttle must cross the net with enough force to carry it as far as the two squares before it touches the floor. If it does not go that far or is outside the space between the two squares, the player being tested should not play it. The player being tested may move any place he wishes as soon as the shuttle has been hit to him. Only shuttles played by the player being tested count as trials. The player attempts to send the shuttle by means of a clear stroke above the rope so that the shuttle lands on the target. Twenty trials are allowed. The person giving the test should call out the score of each trial, to be recorded by an assistant. The area between the two rear lines of the regulation court counts 5 points, the space just behind it counts 3 points, and the space just in front of the two rear lines of the regulation court counts 4 points. Any shuttle going over the rope but failing to reach the target counts 2 points. This test can be given to two players at once on the same court, placing the squares 6 feet from the center line, and each player taking one side of the court.

Scoring

No score is given for any trial failing to go over the rope or failing to land in the court in the space behind the rope and on the target, as

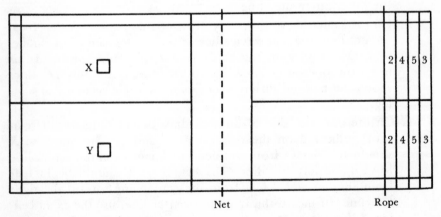

2-5 = scores for respective areas.

x-y = limits of set-up for clear stroke.

Figure 2.22. Floor Markings for Badminton Clear Test.

indicated on the diagram. Any shuttle landing within an area or on the line surrounding the area is scored as shown in the diagram. Any shuttle landing on a line dividing two scoring area receives the score of the higher area. The score for the entire test is the total of twenty trials. It is considered a foul and the trial is repeated if the stroke is "carried" or "slung."

Table 2.29
T-Scales for Badminton Tests

T-Score	Short Serve	Clear	Volleys
80	68	94	
79			
78			
77	67	92	
76			
75		90	148
74	66		
73	64	88	138
72	61		
71	60		128
70	59	86	
69	58	84	114
68	57		110
67	55	82	
66	54	80	
65	53		108
64	52	78	
63	49	76	106
62	48		104
61	46	74	102
60	44	72	100
59	43		98
58	42	70	94
57	41	68	92
56	39	66	90
55	37	64	88
54	36		86
53	35	62	84
52	34	60	
51	31	58	82
50	29	54	
49	28	52	80
48	26	50	78
47	25	48	76
46	23	46	74

T-Score	Short Serve	Clear	Volleys
45	22	44	72
44	21	42	70
43	19	40	68
42	17	38	66
41	15	34	64
40	13	32	62
39	12	30	60
38	11	26	
37	10	24	58
36	9	22	56
35	8	20	54
34	7	18	52
33	6	16	
32	5	12	
31	4	10	50
30		8	48
29		6	46
28	3	4	
27	2		
26			
25	1	2	
24			40
23			
22			
21			

Combinations of Badminton Tests and Multiple Correlations

2.0 wall volley + 1.0 clear + 1.0 short serve.................. .91

2.5 wall volley + 1.0 short serve .... .87

2.0 wall volley + 1.0 clear .... .84

2.0 clear + 1.0 short serve .... .73

BASKETBALL SKILL TESTS*

Front Shot

Purpose

To measure the player's skill in making shots at the basket from a designated spot at the left front of the basket.

*AAHPER, *Basketball Skills Test Manual for Boys and Basketball Skills Test Manual for Girls,* Washington, D.C. American Association for Health, Physical Education, and Recreation, (1201 16th St. N.W., Washington, D.C.). Used by permission of the AAHPER.

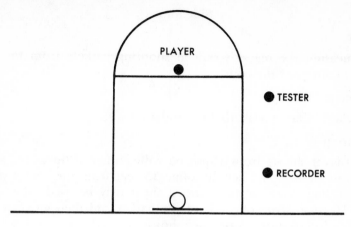

Figure 2.23.

Equipment
Standard inflated basketballs, standard goals.

Description
The player shoots from a spot just outside of the free throw circle where the free throw line intersects the circle. This point is on the left facing the basket. A mark should be drawn on the floor, as in the diagram. Any method of shooting with one or both hands may be used. The player should try to make the shot without hitting the backboard. Fifteen trials are taken in series of five at a time. The player must leave the spot at the end of each five shots and move around or let another player take her first series of shots before continuing. A practice shot is allowed.

Rules
1. Players must shoot from the shooting spot only.
2. Fifteen shots are taken in all.

Scoring
Two points are counted for each basket made, regardless of how the ball goes in. One point is counted for shots which hit the rim but do not go in the basket, provided the ball hits the rim before hitting the backboard. Balls which hit the backboard first and do not go in the basket do not count any points. Record the points as made on each shot, and then total the points for the final score. The maximum score that may be made on the 15 shots is 30 points.

Side Shot

Purpose

To measure the player's skill in shooting baskets from the side, near the corners of the court.

Equipment

Standard inflated basketballs, standard goals.

Description

The player shoots from a spot near the corner of the court, at the side of the basket, and behind a line 15 feet from the center of the basket. Either one— or two-handed shots may be used. The player shoots 10 times from one side of the basket and then moves to the other side for 10 shots. A practice shot is allowed.

Rules

1. Shots must not be taken closer than 15 feet from the basket.

2. Ten shots from each side are taken.

Scoring

Count two points for each goal made and one point for balls which hit the rim of the basket but do not go in, even though they may have hit the backboard also. Score each shot as made and then total the points for the final score. The maximum score possible is 40 points on the 20 shots.

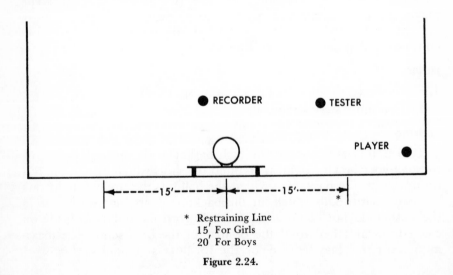

RECORDER   TESTER

PLAYER

|←------15'------→|←------15'------→|
                                   *

* Restraining Line
15' For Girls
20' For Boys

Figure 2.24.

Foul Shot

Purpose

To measure skill in shooting free throws (shooting fouls) from the free throw line.

Equipment

Standard inflated balls, standard goals.

Description

The player shoots from behind the center of the free throw line. The player may shoot by any method preferred. Twenty shots are taken in series of five at a time. The player must leave the foul line at the end of each five shots and move around or let another player take her shots before continuing with her next series of shots. A practice shot is allowed.

Rules

1. Twenty shots are taken in all.

2. The player may place his feet in any position, behind the line.

Scoring

Score one point for each goal made regardless of how the ball goes in. Count each shot as 1 or 0, recording the points in lines of five on the squad score card. Record the total score made. The maximum possible score is 20 points.

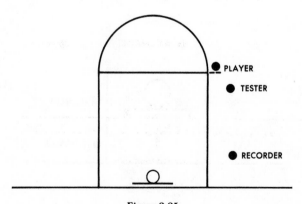

Figure 2.25.

Under Basket Shot

Purpose

To measure skill with which a player can shoot, recover, and shoot from a position directly under the basket.

Equipment

Standard basketball court, standard inflated balls, standard goals, stop watch or watch with sweep-second hand.

Description

The player stands under the basket holding a basketball. On the signal "go" the player starts making one-hand or two-hand lay-up shots, recovering the ball, and shooting again as rapidly as possible, trying to make as many goals as possible within 30 seconds. The player is timed from the signal "go" and is stopped on the signal "stop." A practice trial is allowed.

Rules

1. The ball may be shot in any manner.
2. After shots are made or missed the player recovers the ball and continues shooting.
3. If the player loses the ball entirely, she may start over again, but only once.
4. Two complete trials are allowed.

Scoring

One point is scored for each basket made. The score on the test is the number of baskets made in 30 seconds. Two trials are recorded on the squad card, and the best trial is the player's score.

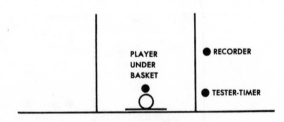

Figure 2.26.

Speed Pass

Purpose

To measure speed with which a player can continue to pass and catch a ball.

Equipment

A level floor or ground and a wall with smooth surface, stop watch, standard inflated basketballs.

Description

The player stands behind a line on the floor parallel to and 9 feet from a solid smooth wall. On the signal "go" the player passes the ball against the wall, about head high, catches the rebound, and continues passing against the wall as rapidly as possible until ten passes have hit the wall. Any method of passing may be used, but the push pass is fastest. A practice trial is allowed.

Rules

1. All passes must be made from behind the line.
2. The ball cannot be batted, but must be caught and passed.
3. The ball can hit the wall at any height.
4. If the ball is dropped, the player must recover it and continue from behind the line until she has hit the wall ten times.
5. Two complete trials are allowed.

Scoring

The test is timed from the instant the first pass hits the wall until the tenth pass hits the wall (the player starts on the signal "go," but the watch is not started until the ball hits the wall). Record the time in seconds and tenths. Two complete trials should be recorded. The score is the best time required to complete ten passes against the wall.

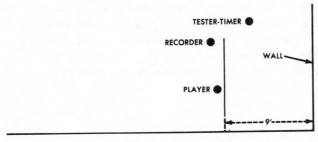

Figure 2.27.

Jump and Reach

Purpose

To measure the height of a player's jump over and above her reach.

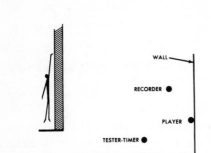

Figure 2.28.

Equipment

A level floor and a smooth wall surface upon which chalk marks can be made, pieces of chalk three-fourth inches long, yard stick. (Some schools may have a prepared target for the jump and reach test, which can be used.)

Description

The player, holding a small piece of chalk in her fingers, stands with her side to the wall with knees straight and feet flat on the floor. She reaches up as far as possible and makes a mark on the wall at the top of her reach. The player then crouches, swings her arms, jumps as high as possible, and makes a second mark on the wall. The distance between the first and second marks on the wall is measured with a yard stick to the nearest inch. A practice jump is allowed.

Rules

1. The player must stand flat-footed with knees straight in making the first mark.
2. The jump must be made from both feet without a hop.
3. Two trials are taken.

Scoring

The score is the distance between the mark at the top of the reach and the mark at the top of the jump. Yard stick must be perpendicular to the floor when measuring the distance between marks. Record the distance to the nearest inch. The distance of the jump on two separate trials is recorded. The score is the best of the two trials.

Overarm Pass For Accuracy

Purpose

To measure the accuracy with which a player can make a single overarm pass at a target.

Equipment

Standard inflated basketballs; a target painted or marked on a wall or on a mat, or on a piece of canvas hung on a smooth wall; chalk, measuring tape. The floor should be properly measured and marked, as in the diagram.

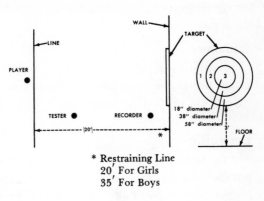

* Restraining Line
20' For Girls
35' For Boys

Figure 2.29.

Description

The player, with a basketball, stands behind a line parallel to and 20 feet from the target marked or hung on a wall. The player throws the ball single overarm at the target. The target is circular with three concentric circles separated by one-inch wide white or black lines. The inner circle is 18 inches in diameter, the next circle is 38 inches in diameter, and the outer circle is 58 inches in diameter. The bottom of the outer circle is 3 feet above the floor. A practice pass is allowed.

Rules

1. The ball can be held in both hands prior to the throw.
2. The throw must be made from behind the line.
3. The player may take a step in throwing, but both feet must be behind the throwing line.
4. Ten passes are taken.

Scoring

Three points are scored for balls hitting in the center circle, two points for balls hitting in the next circle, and one point for balls hitting in the outer circle. Balls hitting on a line count as hitting in the area of the higher score. Points as made on each throw should be recorded, and the total is the score. The maximum possible score is 30 points made on ten passes at the target.

Push Pass For Accuracy

Purpose

To measure accuracy with which a player can make a two-hand push pass at a target.

Equipment

Standard inflated basketballs; a target painted or marked on a wall or on a mat, or on a piece of canvas hung on a smooth wall; chalk; measuring tape. The floor should be properly measured and marked, as in the diagram.

Description

The player with a basketball stands behind a line 15 feet from and parallel to the face of the target marked or hung on a wall. The player uses a two-hand push pass (chest pass) and endeavors to hit the center of the target. The target is the same as used for the overarm pass in Test #7. A practice pass is allowed.

Rules

1. Passes must be made with both feet behind the passing line.
2. The two-hand push, or chest, pass must be used.
3. Ten passes are taken.

Scoring

Three points are scored for balls hitting in the center circle, two points for balls hitting in the next circle, and one point for balls hitting in the outer circle. Hits on a line count as in the next higher area. Points as made on each pass should be recorded, and the total is the score. The maximum possible score is 30 points made on ten passes at the target.

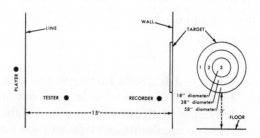

Figure 2.30.

Dribble

Purpose

To measure the speed with which a player can dribble a ball around obstacles.

Equipment

Standard inflated basketballs, stop watch, six chairs arranged as in the diagram.

Description

The player stands behind the starting line with a ball in hand and on the signal "go" starts with a dribble on the right of the first chair and continues to dribble in and out alternately around the remaining five chairs and returns to cross the starting line. The chairs are arranged single file in a straight line so that the front of the first chair is 5 feet from the starting line and the following chairs are 8 feet apart, measured from the front of each chair. All chairs have backs toward the starting line. The over-all distance from the starting line to the far edge of the sixth chair is 45 feet. A practice trial is allowed.

Rules

1. The ball may be dribbled with either hand.
2. Legal dribbles must be used.
3. The ball must be dribbled at least once as each chair is passed, but need not be dribbled opposite a chair.
4. Each player is allowed two trials.

Scoring

The score is the time in seconds and tenths that it takes to dribble around between the chairs and back. Time is started on the signal "go" and stopped the instant the player crosses the starting line at the end of the trip. Two trials are timed and recorded. The best time of the two trials is the player's score on the test.

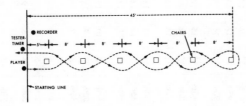

Figure 2.31.

Table 2.30

FRONT SHOT (BOYS)
Percentile Scores Based on Age / Test Scores in Points

Percentile	AGE								Percentile
	10	11	12	13	14	15	16	17-18	
100th	23	26	27	27	27	29	29	30	100th
95th	17	17	18	21	22	22	22	24	95th
90th	15	16	18	19	20	21	21	22	90th
85th	13	15	17	18	20	20	20	21	85th
80th	12	14	16	17	19	20	20	20	80th
75th	11	13	15	16	18	19	19	19	75th
70th	10	12	14	16	17	18	18	18	70th
65th	9	12	14	15	17	17	17	18	65th
60th	9	11	13	15	16	17	17	17	60th
55th	8	10	12	14	16	16	16	17	55th
50th	7	9	11	14	15	16	16	16	50th
45th	7	9	11	13	15	15	15	16	45th
40th	6	8	10	12	14	15	15	15	40th
35th	5	7	9	12	13	14	14	14	35th
30th	4	6	9	11	12	14	14	14	30th
25th	4	6	8	10	12	13	13	13	25th
20th	3	5	7	10	11	12	12	12	20th
15th	2	4	6	8	10	11	11	11	15th
10th	1	2	5	7	9	10	10	10	10th
5th	0	1	3	5	7	7	8	8	5th
0	0	0	0	0	0	3	3	3	0

FRONT SHOT (GIRLS)
Percentile Scores Based on Age / Test Scores in Points

Percentile	AGE							Percentile
	10-11	12	13	14	15	16	17-18	
100th	21	21	30	30	30	30	30	100th
95th	14	15	17	18	18	18	18	95th
90th	12	13	15	16	16	17	17	90th
85th	11	12	14	15	15	15	16	85th
80th	10	11	13	14	14	14	15	80th
75th	9	10	12	13	13	14	14	75th
70th	8	9	11	12	13	13	13	70th
65th	7	9	10	11	12	12	13	65th
60th	6	8	9	10	11	12	12	60th
55th	6	8	9	9	10	11	11	55th
50th	5	7	8	9	9	10	11	50th
45th	4	6	7	8	9	9	10	45th
40th	3	6	6	8	8	9	9	40th
35th	3	5	6	7	7	8	9	35th
30th	2	4	6	6	7	8	8	30th
25th	1	4	5	5	6	7	7	25th
20th	1	3	4	4	5	6	6	20th
15th	1	2	3	3	4	5	5	15th
10th	0	1	2	2	3	4	4	10th
5th	0	0	1	1	2	2	3	5th
0	0	0	0	0	0	0	0	0

Table 2.31

SIDE SHOT (BOYS)
Percentile Scores Based on Age / Test Scores in Points

Percentile	10	11	12	13	14	15	16	17-18	Percentile
100th	27	29	32	33	35	35	35	36	100th
95th	17	18	21	25	26	26	26	26	95th
90th	14	16	20	21	24	24	25	25	90th
85th	13	14	17	20	22	22	22	24	85th
80th	11	13	17	19	21	21	21	22	80th
75th	9	12	15	17	20	20	20	21	75th
70th	8	11	14	16	19	19	19	21	70th
65th	7	10	13	15	18	18	18	20	65th
60th	6	9	12	14	17	17	17	19	60th
55th	5	8	12	14	16	16	16	18	55th
50th	5	7	11	13	16	16	16	18	50th
45th	4	6	10	12	15	15	15	17	45th
40th	3	5	9	11	15	15	15	16	40th
35th	3	5	8	10	14	14	14	15	35th
30th	2	4	7	9	13	13	13	14	30th
25th	1	3	6	8	12	12	12	13	25th
20th	1	2	5	7	11	11	11	12	20th
15th	0	2	4	6	10	10	10	11	15th
10th	0	2	3	5	7	7	9	9	10th
5th	0	2	2	3	5	5	7	7	5th
0	0	0	0	1	1	2	2	2	0

SIDE SHOT (GIRLS)
Percentile Scores Based on Age / Test Scores in Points

Percentile	10-11	12	13	14	15	16	17-18	Percentile
100th	25	26	29	30	31	31	32	100th
95th	16	16	19	21	22	23	22	95th
90th	13	15	17	18	20	20	20	90th
85th	12	13	15	17	18	18	18	85th
80th	11	12	14	16	17	17	17	80th
75th	9	11	13	15	16	16	16	75th
70th	8	10	12	14	15	15	15	70th
65th	7	9	11	13	14	14	14	65th
60th	6	8	11	12	13	13	13	60th
55th	5	7	10	12	12	12	12	55th
50th	4	6	9	11	12	12	12	50th
45th	4	6	8	10	11	11	11	45th
40th	3	5	7	9	10	10	10	40th
35th	2	4	6	8	9	9	9	35th
30th	1	3	6	8	8	8	8	30th
25th	1	3	5	7	7	7	7	25th
20th	0	2	4	6	6	6	6	20th
15th	0	1	3	5	5	5	5	15th
10th	0	0	1	3	3	3	3	10th
5th	0	0	0	1	2	1	1	5th
0	0	0	0	0	0	0	0	0

Table 2.32

FOUL SHOT (BOYS)

Percentile Scores Based on Age / Test Scores in Number of Baskets Made

Percentile	10	11	12	13	14	15	16	17-18	Percentile
100th	13	16	17	20	20	20	20	20	100th
95th	7	8	10	12	13	16	16	16	95th
90th	5	7	8	10	11	13	13	13	90th
85th	4	6	7	9	10	12	12	12	85th
80th	4	5	7	8	10	11	11	11	80th
75th	3	5	6	7	9	10	10	10	75th
70th	3	4	6	7	8	9	9	9	70th
65th	3	4	5	6	8	8	8	9	65th
60th	2	3	5	6	7	8	8	8	60th
55th	2	3	4	5	7	8	8	8	55th
50th	2	3	4	5	6	8	8	8	50th
45th	2	3	4	5	6	7	7	7	45th
40th	1	2	3	4	5	7	7	7	40th
35th	1	2	3	4	5	6	6	6	35th
30th	1	1	3	3	4	5	5	5	30th
25th	0	1	2	3	4	5	5	5	25th
20th	0	1	2	2	4	4	4	4	20th
15th	0	1	1	2	3	4	4	4	15th
10th	0	0	0	1	2	3	3	3	10th
5th	0	0	0	1	2	2	2	2	5th
0	0	0	0	0	0	0	0	0	0

FOUL SHOT (GIRLS)

Percentile Scores Based on Age / Test Scores in Number of Baskets Made

Percentile	10-11	12	13	14	15	16	17-18	Percentile
100th	20	20	20	20	20	20	20	100th
95th	7	8	9	9	9	10	10	95th
90th	5	6	7	7	8	9	9	90th
85th	4	5	6	6	7	8	8	85th
80th	4	5	5	5	6	7	7	80th
75th	3	4	5	5	6	6	6	75th
70th	3	4	4	4	5	6	6	70th
65th	2	3	4	4	5	5	5	65th
60th	2	3	3	3	4	5	5	60th
55th	2	2	3	3	4	4	5	55th
50th	1	2	3	3	4	4	4	50th
45th	1	2	2	3	3	4	4	45th
40th	1	2	2	2	3	3	4	40th
35th	0	1	2	2	3	3	3	35th
30th	0	1	1	2	2	3	3	30th
25th	0	1	1	2	2	2	3	25th
20th	0	1	1	1	2	2	2	20th
15th	0	0	1	1	1	1	2	15th
10th	0	0	0	1	1	1	2	10th
5th	0	0	0	0	0	0	1	5th
0	0	0	0	0	0	0	0	0

Table 2.33

UNDER BASKET SHOT (BOYS)

Percentile Scores Based on Age / Test Scores in Number of Baskets Made

Percentile	10	11	12	13	14	15	16	17-18	Percentile
100th	14	23	23	23	23	29	33	34	100th
95th	10	11	13	15	16	18	19	20	95th
90th	9	10	11	13	15	17	17	18	90th
85th	7	9	10	12	14	16	17	17	85th
80th	7	8	10	12	14	15	15	16	80th
75th	6	8	9	11	13	15	15	15	75th
70th	6	7	9	10	12	14	14	15	70th
65th	6	6	8	10	12	13	14	14	65th
60th	5	6	8	9	11	13	13	14	60th
55th	5	6	7	9	11	13	13	14	55th
50th	5	5	7	8	10	11	12	13	50th
45th	4	5	7	8	10	11	12	12	45th
40th	4	5	5	6	9	10	11	11	40th
35th	4	4	5	6	9	9	10	11	35th
30th	3	4	5	6	8	9	9	10	30th
25th	3	4	4	5	8	8	9	10	25th
20th	3	3	4	5	7	8	8	9	20th
15th	2	3	4	5	6	7	7	8	15th
10th	2	2	3	3	4	6	6	7	10th
5th	1	1	2	2	3	4	5	6	5th
0	0	1	1	1	1	1	1	1	0

UNDER BASKET SHOT (GIRLS)

Percentile Scores Based on Age / Test Scores in Number of Baskets Made

Percentile	10-11	12	13	14	15	16	17-18	Percentile
100th	15	15	16	16	18	19	20	100th
95th	8	10	10	11	11	13	13	95th
90th	7	8	8	10	10	11	11	90th
85th	6	7	8	9	9	10	10	85th
80th	5	7	7	8	8	9	9	80th
75th	5	6	7	8	8	8	8	75th
70th	5	6	7	7	7	8	8	70th
65th	5	5	6	7	7	7	7	65th
60th	4	5	6	6	6	7	7	60th
55th	4	5	6	6	6	6	6	55th
50th	4	4	5	6	6	6	6	50th
45th	4	4	5	5	5	5	5	45th
40th	3	4	5	5	5	5	5	40th
35th	3	4	4	5	5	5	5	35th
30th	3	3	4	4	4	4	4	30th
25th	2	3	4	4	4	4	4	25th
20th	2	3	3	4	4	4	4	20th
15th	2	2	3	3	3	3	3	15th
10th	1	2	2	3	3	3	3	10th
5th	1	1	1	2	2	2	2	5th
0	0	0	0	1	1	1	1	0

103

Table 2.34

SPEED PASS (BOYS)

Percentile Scores Based on Age / Test Scores in Seconds and Tenths

Percentile	10	11	12	13	14	15	16	17-18	Percentile
100th	10.0	8.5	5.5	5.5	5.5	4.5	4.5	4.5	100th
95th	11.6	10.5	8.5	7.8	7.6	7.4	7.3	6.8	95th
90th	11.6	11.2	9.7	8.3	8.0	7.8	7.7	7.2	90th
85th	12.2	11.6	10.1	8.8	8.3	8.0	7.9	7.5	85th
80th	12.5	11.9	10.4	9.3	8.6	8.3	8.1	7.8	80th
75th	12.8	12.2	10.7	9.8	8.9	8.5	8.4	8.0	75th
70th	13.1	12.4	11.1	10.0	9.0	8.7	8.6	8.2	70th
65th	13.3	12.7	11.4	10.3	9.2	8.9	8.7	8.3	65th
60th	13.6	12.9	11.7	10.6	9.4	9.1	8.9	8.6	60th
55th	13.9	13.2	11.7	10.8	9.6	9.3	9.1	8.8	55th
50th	14.2	13.4	12.2	11.1	9.9	9.4	9.2	9.0	50th
45th	14.6	13.7	12.5	11.4	10.2	9.6	9.4	9.2	45th
40th	14.9	14.0	12.7	11.8	10.4	10.0	9.6	9.4	40th
35th	15.2	14.3	13.0	12.2	10.6	10.2	9.9	9.6	35th
30th	15.6	14.6	13.3	12.6	11.0	10.5	10.2	9.9	30th
25th	16.0	14.9	13.6	13.0	11.3	10.9	10.5	10.2	25th
20th	16.5	15.3	14.2	13.4	11.7	11.3	11.1	10.5	20th
15th	17.3	15.7	14.9	14.2	12.2	12.0	11.6	11.1	15th
10th	18.1	16.3	15.5	15.1	13.0	12.8	12.5	11.9	10th
5th	19.3	17.5	16.9	16.6	14.4	14.1	14.0	13.4	5th
0	26.0	26.5	25.0	21.4	20.4	20.4	20.3	20.0	0

SPEED PASS (GIRLS)

Percentile Scores Based on Age / Test Scores in Seconds and Tenths

Percentile	10-11	12	13	14	15	16	17-18	Percentile
100th	7.5	7.5	7.5	7.5	7.5	6.5	6.5	100th
95th	11.9	10.5	10.4	10.0	9.5	9.5	9.5	95th
90th	12.6	11.1	11.1	10.7	10.2	10.1	10.0	90th
85th	12.9	11.7	11.7	11.1	10.7	10.6	10.4	85th
80th	13.2	12.0	12.0	11.5	11.0	10.9	10.7	80th
75th	13.5	12.4	12.4	11.8	11.3	11.2	11.0	75th
70th	13.9	12.8	12.7	12.1	11.6	11.5	11.3	70th
65th	14.2	13.1	13.0	12.4	11.9	11.8	11.6	65th
60th	14.5	13.4	13.2	12.7	12.2	12.1	11.9	60th
55th	14.9	13.7	13.5	13.0	12.5	12.4	12.2	55th
50th	15.3	14.0	13.8	13.4	12.8	12.7	12.5	50th
45th	15.6	14.4	14.2	13.7	13.1	13.0	12.8	45th
40th	15.9	14.8	14.5	14.0	13.5	13.4	13.1	40th
35th	16.3	15.1	14.9	14.4	13.9	13.6	13.4	35th
30th	16.7	15.5	15.3	14.8	14.3	14.1	13.8	30th
25th	17.2	16.1	15.8	15.1	14.8	14.5	14.4	25th
20th	17.7	16.8	16.4	15.5	15.3	15.1	15.0	20th
15th	18.3	17.6	17.1	16.2	16.1	15.7	15.7	15th
10th	19.1	18.4	18.2	17.3	17.0	16.6	16.6	10th
5th	20.3	21.1	20.0	19.2	18.6	18.0	17.9	5th
0	25.5	25.4	25.4	25.4	25.4	25.4	24.4	0

Table 2.35

JUMP AND REACH (BOYS)
Percentile Scores Based on Age / Test Scores in Inches

Percentile	10	11	12	13	14	15	16	17-18	Percentile
100th	18	22	25	29	29	31	31	34	100th
95th	14	16	18	20	22	24	24	26	95th
90th	13	15	17	19	21	22	23	25	90th
85th	13	14	16	18	21	21	22	24	85th
80th	12	14	16	17	20	21	21	24	80th
75th	12	13	15	17	19	20	21	23	75th
70th	12	13	15	17	19	20	21	23	70th
65th	11	12	14	16	18	19	20	22	65th
60th	11	12	14	16	18	19	20	22	60th
55th	11	12	13	15	17	18	19	21	55th
50th	10	11	13	15	17	18	19	20	50th
45th	10	11	13	14	16	17	18	20	45th
40th	10	11	13	14	16	17	18	19	40th
35th	10	10	12	14	15	17	18	19	35th
30th	9	10	12	13	15	16	17	18	30th
25th	9	10	11	13	14	16	17	18	25th
20th	9	9	10	11	13	14	15	16	20th
15th	8	9	10	11	13	14	14	15	15th
10th	8	8	10	11	13	13	14	15	10th
5th	6	7	9	9	12	12	13	14	5th
0	4	4	5	5	7	7	8	13	0

JUMP AND REACH (GIRLS)
Percentile Scores Based on Age / Test Scores in Inches

Percentile	10-11	12	13	14	15	16	17-18	Percentile
100th	18	21	24	24	25	25	25	100th
95th	15	16	17	18	18	18	18	95th
90th	14	15	16	16	17	17	17	90th
85th	13	14	15	15	16	16	16	85th
80th	12	14	15	15	16	16	16	80th
75th	12	13	14	14	15	15	15	75th
70th	11	13	14	14	15	15	15	70th
65th	11	13	13	14	14	14	14	65th
60th	11	12	13	13	14	14	14	60th
55th	10	12	12	13	14	14	14	55th
50th	10	12	12	13	13	13	13	50th
45th	10	11	12	12	13	13	13	45th
40th	10	11	11	12	13	13	13	40th
35th	9	11	11	12	12	12	12	35th
30th	9	10	11	11	12	12	12	30th
25th	9	10	10	11	11	11	12	25th
20th	9	9	10	10	11	11	11	20th
15th	8	9	9	10	10	10	11	15th
10th	8	9	9	9	10	10	10	10th
5th	7	8	8	9	9	9	9	5th
0	5	5	5	5	7	7	7	0

Table 2.36

OVERARM PASS FOR ACCURACY (BOYS)
Percentile Scores Based on Age / Test Scores in Points

Percentile	AGE								Percentile
	10	11	12	13	14	15	16	17-18	
100th	18	27	27	27	29	31	31	31	100th
95th	14	18	20	20	22	24	24	25	95th
90th	13	15	18	19	21	22	22	23	90th
85th	11	14	17	18	20	21	21	22	85th
80th	10	12	16	17	19	20	20	21	80th
75th	8	11	15	16	18	19	19	20	75th
70th	7	11	14	16	18	19	19	19	70th
65th	6	10	13	15	17	17	18	18	65th
60th	6	9	12	15	17	17	17	17	60th
55th	5	8	12	14	16	17	17	17	55th
50th	4	7	11	13	16	16	16	16	50th
45th	3	6	10	12	15	15	15	15	45th
40th	2	5	10	12	14	15	15	15	40th
35th	2	4	9	11	14	14	14	14	35th
30th	1	3	8	10	13	13	13	13	30th
25th	0	2	7	9	12	12	12	12	25th
20th	0	2	6	9	10	11	11	11	20th
15th	0	1	5	8	10	10	11	11	15th
10th	0	0	3	6	9	9	9	9	10th
5th	0	0	2	4	7	7	8	8	5th
0	0	0	0	0	0	0	0	2	0

OVERARM PASS FOR ACCURACY (GIRLS)
Percentile Scores Based on Age / Test Scores in Points

Percentile	AGE							Percentile
	10-11	12	13	14	15	16	17-18	
100th	27	29	30	30	30	30	30	100th
95th	23	24	25	25	26	26	26	95th
90th	22	23	24	24	25	25	25	90th
85th	21	22	23	23	24	24	24	85th
80th	19	21	22	22	23	23	23	80th
75th	18	20	21	21	22	22	22	75th
70th	17	19	20	20	22	22	22	70th
65th	16	18	19	20	21	21	21	65th
60th	14	17	18	19	20	21	20	60th
55th	13	16	18	18	20	20	19	55th
50th	12	15	17	18	19	19	19	50th
45th	11	15	17	17	18	18	18	45th
40th	10	14	15	16	17	17	17	40th
35th	8	13	14	15	17	17	15	35th
30th	7	12	13	15	16	16	14	30th
25th	5	11	12	14	15	15	13	25th
20th	4	9	11	13	13	14	11	20th
15th	2	7	9	11	12	12	10	15th
10th	0	4	7	9	9	9	8	10th
5th	0	1	4	6	6	6	5	5th
0	0	0	0	0	0	0	0	0

Table 2.37

PUSH PASS FOR ACCURACY (BOYS)
Percentile Scores Based on Age / Test Scores in Points

Percentile	11	12	13	14	15	16	17-18	Percentile
100th	29	29	29	29	29	30	30	100th
95th	19	22	24	25	27	27	29	95th
90th	17	20	22	24	25	26	28	90th
85th	14	18	21	23	24	25	28	85th
80th	12	16	20	21	23	24	27	80th
75th	11	14	19	21	23	23	27	75th
70th	9	13	18	20	22	23	26	70th
65th	8	12	17	19	21	22	26	65th
60th	7	11	16	18	21	21	26	60th
55th	5	10	15	18	20	21	25	55th
50th	4	9	13	17	19	20	24	50th
45th	3	8	13	16	19	19	24	45th
40th	2	7	12	15	18	18	23	40th
35th	1	5	11	14	17	18	23	35th
30th	1	4	10	14	16	17	22	30th
25th	1	3	9	12	15	16	21	25th
20th	1	2	7	11	14	15	20	20th
15th	0	2	5	10	13	14	18	15th
10th	0	1	2	8	11	12	17	10th
5th	0	1	1	4	6	9	14	5th
0	0	0	1	1	2	4	5	0

NOTE: This test has proved too difficult for ten-year-old boys at the distance used, and hence scores for boys age ten are omitted from this table.

PUSH PASS FOR ACCURACY (GIRLS)
Percentile Scores Based on Age / Test Scores in Points

Percentile	10-11	12	13	14	15	16	17-18	Percentile
100th	29	30	30	30	30	30	30	100th
95th	26	27	28	28	29	29	29	95th
90th	24	26	27	28	28	28	28	90th
85th	23	25	26	27	27	27	27	85th
80th	22	24	25	26	27	27	27	80th
75th	21	23	24	25	26	26	26	75th
70th	21	22	24	25	25	26	26	70th
65th	20	22	23	24	25	25	25	65th
60th	19	21	22	23	24	25	25	60th
55th	18	20	22	23	24	24	24	55th
50th	17	19	21	22	23	24	24	50th
45th	16	19	21	22	23	23	23	45th
40th	15	18	20	21	22	22	23	40th
35th	13	17	19	20	22	22	22	35th
30th	12	16	18	19	21	21	21	30th
25th	10	14	17	18	20	20	20	25th
20th	8	12	15	17	19	19	19	20th
15th	7	10	13	15	18	17	17	15th
10th	4	8	11	13	16	12	13	10th
5th	2	4	7	10	12	8	9	5th
0	0	0	0	0	0	0	0	0

Table 2.38

DRIBBLING (GIRLS)

Percentile Scores Based on Age / Test Scores in Seconds and Tenths

Percentile	AGE							Percentile
	10-11	12	13	14	15	16	17-18	
100th	9.5	9.5	9.5	9.5	9.5	8.5	7.5	100th
95th	13.7	12.0	11.7	11.7	11.7	10.9	10.8	95th
90th	14.5	12.9	12.8	12.6	12.3	11.7	11.7	90th
85th	14.9	13.5	13.3	13.0	12.8	12.1	12.0	85th
80th	15.2	14.0	13.7	13.4	13.1	12.5	12.4	80th
75th	15.6	14.3	14.0	13.7	13.4	12.7	12.7	75th
70th	15.9	14.6	14.4	14.0	13.6	13.0	13.0	70th
65th	16.2	14.9	14.7	14.3	13.8	13.2	13.2	65th
60th	16.5	15.2	14.9	14.5	14.0	13.5	13.4	60th
55th	16.8	15.5	15.1	14.8	14.2	13.7	13.6	55th
50th	17.1	15.8	15.4	15.0	14.5	14.0	14.0	50th
45th	17.5	16.2	15.7	15.2	14.7	14.3	14.3	45th
40th	17.8	16.5	16.1	15.5	15.0	14.6	14.5	40th
35th	18.2	16.9	16.4	15.8	15.3	14.9	14.7	35th
30th	18.5	17.3	16.7	16.2	15.6	15.2	15.0	30th
25th	19.0	17.7	17.1	16.5	16.0	15.5	15.2	25th
20th	19.5	18.2	17.5	17.0	16.3	16.0	15.5	20th
15th	20.4	18.7	18.0	17.5	16.9	16.5	16.3	15th
10th	21.1	20.5	18.2	17.8	17.2	17.1	17.0	10th
5th	22.4	21.2	20.6	19.8	18.9	18.4	18.0	5th
0	29.0	24.5	24.5	24.5	24.5	24.5	24.5	0

DRIBBLING (BOYS)

Percentile Scores Based on Age / Test Scores in Seconds and Tenths

Percentile	AGE								Percentile
	10	11	12	13	14	15	16	17-18	
100th	12.0	10.5	6.5	6.5	6.5	5.5	5.5	5.5	100th
95th	13.0	12.0	10.3	9.8	9.7	9.5	9.5	8.8	95th
90th	13.7	12.8	11.3	10.4	10.1	9.8	9.8	9.5	90th
85th	14.1	13.0	11.7	10.8	10.7	10.1	10.0	9.9	85th
80th	14.6	13.3	12.1	11.2	10.9	10.3	10.3	10.3	80th
75th	14.8	13.6	12.3	11.6	11.1	10.6	10.5	10.5	75th
70th	15.1	13.9	12.6	11.9	11.3	10.9	10.8	10.8	70th
65th	15.3	14.1	12.9	12.2	11.5	11.1	11.0	11.0	65th
60th	15.5	14.4	13.2	12.4	11.8	11.4	11.3	11.2	60th
55th	15.8	14.7	13.4	12.7	12.0	11.7	11.5	11.5	55th
50th	16.0	15.0	13.7	13.0	12.3	12.0	11.8	11.7	50th
45th	16.3	15.3	14.1	13.3	12.6	12.3	12.1	11.8	45th
40th	16.5	15.6	14.4	13.6	12.9	12.6	12.3	12.0	40th
35th	16.9	16.0	14.7	13.9	13.2	12.9	12.6	12.3	35th
30th	17.2	16.3	15.0	14.2	13.6	13.2	12.9	12.6	30th
25th	17.6	16.8	15.3	14.4	13.9	13.5	13.2	13.0	25th
20th	18.0	17.2	15.8	14.9	14.3	14.0	13.4	13.3	20th
15th	18.4	17.9	16.5	15.3	14.8	14.5	13.8	13.7	15th
10th	19.4	18.8	17.3	16.1	15.6	15.2	14.2	14.2	10th
5th	21.4	20.4	18.7	18.3	17.4	16.5	14.7	14.6	5th
0	26.0	26.5	26.5	23.0	22.0	22.0	21.6	21.5	0

108

FIELD HOCKEY SKILL TESTS*

DESCRIPTION OF TESTS

Test One: Dribble, Dodge, Circular Tackle, and Drive

Equipment.—

1. Hockey stick for each participant.
2. Stop watch, checked by a jeweler.
3. One ball necessary; two balls convenient.
4. High jump standards.
5. Field markings (see Figure 2.32).
   a. A line 20 feet long to be used for a starting line.
   b. A line perpendicular to the midpoint of the starting line and extending 35 feet from it. This is the foul line.
   c. A line 10 feet long, perpendicular to and being bisected by the foul line at a point 30 feet from the starting line. This is the restraining line.
   d. A line 1 foot long, perpendicular to and being bisected by the foul line at a point 35 feet from the starting line.
   e. Two lines, each 1 foot long, bisecting each other at a point which is 45 feet from the starting line and in a straight line with the foul line.
6. Position of standards:
   a. One standard is placed so that the middle of the base of the standard is directly over the point where the foul line and the line described in 5d bisect each other.
   b. The other standard is placed in similar fashion over the point formed by the two lines described in 5c.

*Test.—*The player being tested shall stand behind the starting line with the hockey ball placed on the starting line at any point to the left of the foul line. At the signal "Ready? Go!" the player shall dribble the ball forward to the left of and parallel to the foul line. As soon as the restraining line is reached, the ball shall be sent from the left side of the foul line to the right of the first obstacle (from the player's point of view), and the player shall run around the left side of the obstacle and recover the ball. (This is analogous to a dodge.) Next, the player shall execute a turn toward her right around the

---

*Schmithals, Margaret and Esther French, "Achievement Tests in Field Hockey for College Women," *Research Quarterly,* 11, 84-92, October, 1940. Used by permission of the AAHPER.

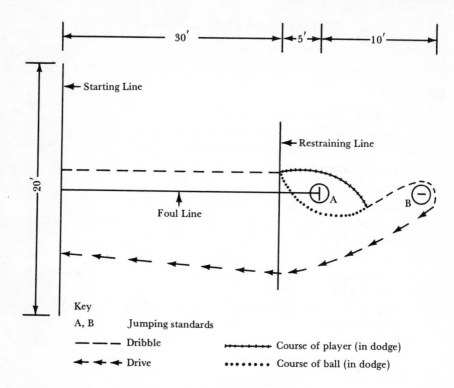

Figure 2.32. Field Markings for Test One.

second obstacle, still keeping control of the ball. (This is analogous to a circular tackle.) As soon as possible after that the ball shall be driven toward the starting line. If the drive is not hard enough to reach the starting line the player may follow it up and hit the ball again.

This procedure shall be repeated until six trials have been given, care being taken that no player is fatigued.

Scoring.—The score for one trial shall be the time it takes from the signal "Go" until the player's ball has again crossed the starting line. The score for the entire test is the average of the six trials. It is considered a foul and the trial does not count if:

1. The ball or player crosses the foul line before reaching the restraining line.
2. In executing the dodge, the ball is not sent from the left side of the foul line.
3. The player makes "sticks."

Test Two: Goal Shooting—Straight, Right, Left

Equipment.—

1. Target, 9 inches wide, 12 feet long, and at least 1/2 inch thick, made of hard wood.

The board is painted according to the following specifications: The length of the board is divided into eleven equal spaces, alternate spaces starting from either end being painted black and the other remaining the natural color of the wood. Numbers are painted in the spaces in contrasting colors (black on light background and white on black background) in the following order starting from either end: 1-2-3-4-5-6-5-4-3-2-1 (See Figure 2.34).

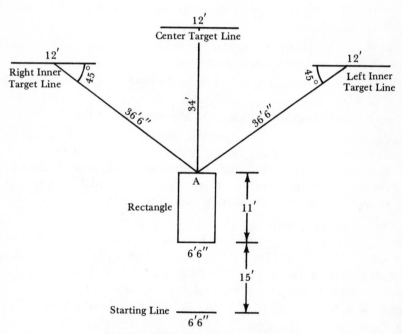

Figure 2.33. Field Markings for Test Two.

A base made of board at least 3 inches wide, exactly 12 feet long, and at least 1/2 inch thick, is nailed on the bottom of the target so that two and one-half inches extend beyond the back of the target. The board, in order to stand upright securely, may be anchored with an ice pick or other similar device.

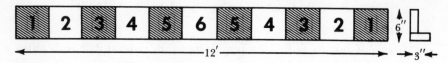

Figure 2.34. Front and Side Views of Target for Test Two.

2. Same as *1* and *2* in test one.

3. At least four balls necessary; ten balls convenient.

4. Field markings (See Figure 2.33):

a. A line 6 feet 6 inches long to be used for a starting line.

b. A rectangle 11 feet long and 6 feet 6 inches wide, 15 feet from the starting line. Point A is the midpoint of the side opposite the starting line.

c. A line 12 feet long, called the center target line, parallel to and 60 feet from the starting line.

d. A line 12 feet long, called the right inner target line (See Figure 2.33).

e. A line 12 feet long, called the left inner target line.

5. Position of target: The target is placed directly on the specified line with the numbers facing the starting line and the board anchored with ice picks. For the straight drive, it is placed on the center target line, for the drive from right and left inner's positions, the right and left inner's target lines, respectively.

Test.—1. Drive from the Center's Position. The player being tested shall stand behind the starting line with the hockey ball placed directly on the starting line. At the signal "Ready? Go!" the ball shall be dribbled to the rectangle, from *within which area* it must be driven toward the board (placed on the center target line). This procedure shall be repeated until ten trials have been given.

2. Drive from Right Inner's Position. The same procedure shall be repeated, the only difference being the position of the board, which is placed on the right inner target line.

3. Drive from Left Inner's Position. The same procedure shall be repeated, the only difference being the change in position of the target to the left inner target line.

Scoring.—The score for one trial shall constitute the time elapsing from the timer's signal "Go!" until the ball strikes the board. The score for the entire test is the sum of the first and second best odd and first and second best even numbered scores made on the center drive, the right inner drive, and the left inner drive. The score shall count if the ball bounces over the top of the target. In this case, the time shall be taken until the instant that the ball clears the target. Players shall receive a score of zero on a trial if:

1. The ball is not driven from within the rectangle.
2. The driven ball fails to reach the board or misses it at either end.

The attempt is not counted as a trial if:

1. "Sticks" are made.
2. Player raises the ball so that it doesn't touch the ground before it passes over the target.

Test Three—Fielding and Drive

Equipment.—

1. Same as for *1* and *2* in test one.
2. At least three balls necessary; seven or eight balls convenient.
3. Two ice picks with brightly covered tops.
4. Regulation hockey goal, including goal line and striking circle.
5. Special field markings (See Figure 2.35):
    a. "Goal line" that is referred to is the line between the two goal posts. Midpoint of the goal line is referred to as point *B*.
    b. Foul line, 12 feet long, parallel to and 10 feet from the goal line.
    c. Restraining line, 30 feet long, parallel to and 10 feet from the foul line.
6. Each ice pick is placed on the foul line at a point directly opposite each goal post.

Test.—The player being tested shall stand behind the goal line. The examiner shall stand at the edge of the striking circle directly in front of the goal with a hockey ball in one hand and a stop watch in the other. At the examiner's signal "Ready? Go!" the hockey ball is rolled toward the goal at approximately the speed of 45 feet in 1.7 seconds. Simultaneously, the player shall run forward and attempt to field the ball before it reaches the foul line, tap it once, and drive it out of the striking circle from within the area between the restraining line and the foul line. This procedure shall be repeated until sixteen trials have been given.

Scoring.—The score for one trial is the time from the moment the player first touches the hockey ball to the moment the ball reaches the striking circle. The score on the entire test is the sum of the average of the three best even and three best odd numbered scores of the sixteen trials.

The attempt does not count as a trial if:

1. The rolled ball does not pass between the two ice picks.
2. The rolled ball is not delivered at approximately the speed designated.
3. The player makes "sticks."

The player receives no score on a particular trial if:

1. The ball is advanced illegally.
2. The ball rolls wholly over the foul line before or after it is touched by the player's stick.
3. The ball is not driven out of striking circle from within the area bounded by the restraining line and foul line.
4. The ball is not controlled; that is, stopped, tapped, and driven.

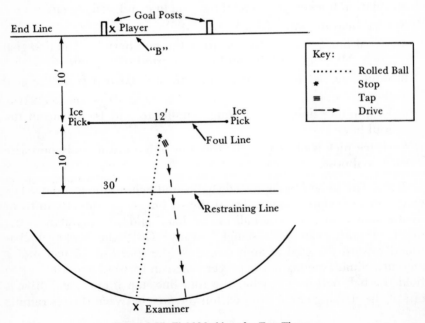

Figure 2.35. Field Markings for Test Three.

FOOTBALL SKILL TESTS*
Forward Pass For Distance

Purpose

To measure the straightaway distance the player can throw a forward pass after taking one or more steps.

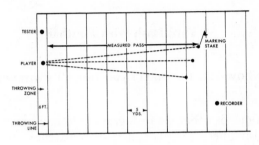

Figure 2.36.

Equipment

A playing field properly marked off for football or some other sports field with throwing lane marked, standard footballs in good condition, measuring tape, wire marking stakes (which can be made from coat hangers).

Description

The player throws a forward pass for distance from between two parallel lines 6 feet apart. The player takes one or more running steps inside this zone and throws as far as possible without stepping over the second line. The first pass is marked by inserting a stake at the point where the ball first hits the ground. If a succeeding pass is longer, the stake is moved to the farther spot. The longest pass is then measured and recorded.

Rules

1. The player must warm up before being tested and is allowed one practice pass.

*AAHPER, *Football Skills Test Manual,* Washington, D.C. American Association for Health, Physical Education, and Recreation, (1201 16th St. N.W., Washington, D.C.). Used by permission of the AAHPER.

2. Passes must be thrown from inside the throwing zone.

3. The player is allowed three passes.

4. Distances must be measured at right angles to the throwing line.

Scoring

The score is the distance in full feet measured to the last foot passed, disregarding inches, from the throwing line to the point where the longest pass hits the ground.

50-Yard Dash With Football

Purpose

To measure how fast the player can run 50 yards with a football.

Equipment

A football field or other smooth grass field laid out with a starting line and a finish line 50 yards apart, stop watches, measuring tape, standard footballs, a white handkerchief or cloth.

Description

The player stands behind the starting line holding a football. The starter stands slightly ahead of the starting line and holds a white handkerchief or cloth in his upraised hand. When the starter simultaneously shouts "go" and vigorously swings down the handkerchief, the player starts. The timer stands on the finish line and starts his watch when the handkerchief swings down. The player runs the 50 yards carrying the ball. The timer stops his watch as the player crosses the finish line. If enough watches and timers are available, two or more players can run at a time, thus providing competition.

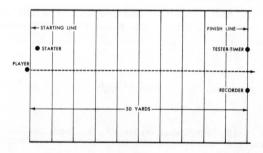

Figure 2.37.

Rules

1. The player must warm up before being tested.
2. The player must carry a football the full distance.
3. The player runs the distance twice, resting in between.

Scoring

The score is the time in seconds and tenths from the starter's arm signal to the instant the runner crosses the finish line. The time of each dash should be noted, and the best time is the player's score.

Blocking

Purpose

To measure the player's speed and agility in executing three cross-body blocks.

Equipment

A football field or other smooth grass field, three blocking bags, measuring tape, stop watch. (For the blocking bags, canvas bags 18 inches in diameter and 4 feet high can be used. They should be filled with sand and closed at the top.)

Description

Set up the course so that the three blocking bags are arranged as shown in the diagram. Place bags 1 and 2 on end 15 feet apart and each 15 feet from the starting line. Place bag 3 on end 15 feet from bag 2 in the direction of the starting line and at a 45-degree angle to the line between bag 1 and bag 2. This will put bag 3 about 5 feet

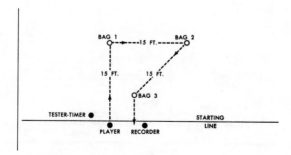

Figure 2.38.

from the starting line. The player stands behind the starting line opposite bag 1, and on the signal "go" he charges forward and cross-body blocks bag 1 clear to the ground. He then recovers immediately, charges across to bag 2, and blocks it clear to the ground. He recovers again, charges back to bag 3, and blocks it to the ground. He then recovers and charges straight across the starting line. The player is timed from the signal "go" to the instant he crosses the starting line after blocking down bag 3.

Rules

1. The player must warm up before being tested and is allowed one practice run-through.
2. Each bag must be cross-body blocked clear to the ground with the player on top. He cannot just bump the bag down.
3. The player is given two trials and each time is recorded.

Scoring

The score is the time in seconds and tenths required for the player to finish the test; time is started on signal "go" and stopped as the player crosses back over the line. The best time is the player's score.

Forward Pass For Accuracy

Purpose

To measure the player's skill in forward passing at a target.

Equipment

Official football goal posts, a large piece of canvas with a target painted on it, a marked throwing line, standard footballs.

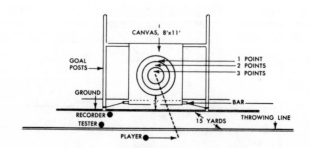

Figure 2.39.

Description

The canvas target is hung from the cross bar of the goal posts. The player stands behind the throwing line, which is 15 yards from and parallel to the goal posts. The player starts opposite the center of the target, takes two or three small running steps along the line, hesitates, and immediately throws at the target. The player may take his steps either to the right or to the left, but he must stay behind the throwing line. The target consists of a sheet of canvas about 8 feet by 11 feet, with three concentric circles painted on it. The center circle is 2 feet in diameter, the middle circle 4 feet in diameter, and the outer circle 6 feet in diameter. Circle lines are one inch wide, in either black or white paint for best contrast. The canvas is hung with the narrow end over the cross bar and tied. The bottom of the outer circle should be exactly 3 feet above the ground. The canvas should have a channel sewed along the bottom, into which a wood or metal bar is inserted; each end should be tied to a goal post to keep the canvas taut.

Rules

1. The player must warm up before being tested and is allowed one practice throw.
2. The player must pass the ball with good speed.
3. The player throws ten passes at the target.
4. Points made on each pass are recorded.

Scoring

Passes hitting within the inner circle area count three points, passes hitting within the middle circle area count two points, and passes hitting in the outer circle area count one point. Passes hitting a line count the higher number of points. The player's score is the total points made for ten throws.

Football Punt For Distance

Purpose

To measure the distance a player can punt a football in a free kick.

Equipment

Regulation football field or smooth grass field with a kicking zone marked, standard inflated footballs, measuring tape, wire marking stakes.

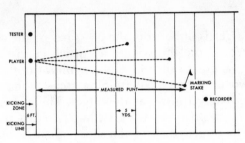

Figure 2.40.

Description

The player stands in the kicking zone behind the kicking line, holding a football. He takes one or two steps inside the zone and punts the ball as far as possible. The first punt is marked by inserting a stake at the point where the ball first hits the ground. If a succeeding punt is longer, the stake is moved to the farther spot.

Rules

1. The player must warm up before being tested and is allowed one practice punt.
2. The player is allowed three punts.
3. The ball must be punted from within the kicking zone.
4. All punts must be measured at right angles to the kicking line.

Scoring

The score is the distance in full feet measured to the last foot passed, disregarding inches, from the kicking line to the point where the longest punt hits the ground.

Ball Changing Zigzag Run

Purpose

To measure a player's speed as he zigzags and changes a football from arm to arm.

Equipment

A football field or other smooth grass field, five chairs (with spares available), standard footballs, stop watch, measuring tape.

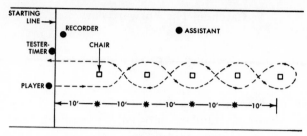

Figure 2.41.

Description

Five chairs are arranged in a line with the first chair 10 feet from the starting line and each succeeding chair 10 feet farther on. All chairs face away from the starting line. The player stands behind the starting line with a football under his right arm. On the signal "go" he runs to the right around the first chair, changes the ball to his left arm as he passes to the left of the second chair, and continues in and out around each chair. He circles around the end chair and then returns in the same manner to the starting line. Each time he goes around a chair he must have the ball under his outside arm and the inside arm must be extended as if for a stiff arm at the chair he is passing. An assistant should inspect the run and report any violations.

Rules

1. The player must warm up before being tested and is allowed one practice run.
2. Each time the player goes around a chair he must have the ball under his outside arm and his inside arm extended toward the chair.
3. The player must not hit the chairs.
4. The player is given two runs and each time is recorded.

Scoring

The score is the time in seconds and tenths of seconds measured from the signal "go" to the instant the player crosses back over the starting line. Two valid runs are timed. The best time is the score on the test.

Catching The Forward Pass

Purpose

To measure a player's ability to catch a spot pass.

Equipment

A football field or other smooth grass field marked for the test as shown in the diagram, standard footballs, measuring tape, baseball bases or white cloths to mark points.

Description

The success of this test depends upon having one or more expert passers who can pass the ball mechanically over the passing point without attention to the player trying to catch the pass. A scrimmage line is laid out. An assistant serves as center over the ball on the scrimmage line. The player being tested takes a position as an end 9 feet from the center on the right. A "turning point" is marked 30 feet directly ahead of the player on the scrimmage line. A "passing point" is marked 30 feet from the turning point to the right and 30 feet from the scrimmage line. A similar turning point and passing point are laid out to the left of the center. The passer stands 15 feet directly behind the center. On the signal "go" the center snaps the ball to the passer, who takes a step and passes the ball directly over the passing point above head height. On the signal "go" the player runs straight ahead around the turning point and out beyond the passing point and tries to catch the ball.

Rules

1. The player must warm up before being tested and is allowed one practice run-through on each side.

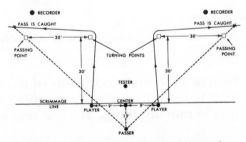

This diagram shows the field markings and action for catching passes from both sides.

Figure 2.42.

2. The player need not try for bad balls.

3. The player must go around the turning point.

4. To be good the pass must go over the passing point.

5. The player is thrown ten passes on each side.

Scoring

One point is scored for each pass caught after the pass has crossed over the passing point. The score is the sum of passes caught from both sides.

Pull-Out

Purpose

To measure the speed with which a player can pull out of a scrimmage line and charge forward a short distance.

Equipment

A football field with standard goal posts, stop watch, measuring tape.

Description

The player takes a set position as if on a scrimmage line with his hands on a line running through the goal posts, halfway between the two posts. On the signal "go" he pulls out of the line and dashes around the right hand goal post and charges straight ahead across a finish line which is 30 feet from and parallel to the line through the goal posts.

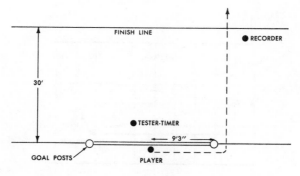

Figure 2.43.

Rules

1. The player must warm up before being tested and is allowed one practice run.
2. The player must face straight ahead.
3. The player must start from the exact center between the goal posts.
4. The player must not move hand or foot until the signal "go."
5. Two trials are given.

Scoring

The score is the time in seconds and tenths of seconds from the signal "go" to the instant the player crosses the finish line. Both trials are timed and recorded. The better of the two times is the player's score.

Kick-Off

Purpose

To measure the distance a player can place-kick a football.

Equipment

A football field or other smooth grass field, a kicking tee, standard footballs, measuring tape, wire marking stakes.

Description

The ball is set up on a kicking tee so that it tilts slightly back toward the kicker. The ball should be set at the center of one of the lines running across the field. The player takes as long a run as he wants and kicks the ball as far as possible. The first kick is marked by

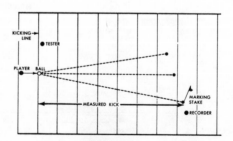

Figure 2.44.

inserting a stake at the point where the ball first hits the ground. If a succeeding kick is longer the stake is moved to the farther spot. The longest kick is then measured and recorded.

Rules

1. The player must warm up before being tested and is allowed one practice kick.
2. The player must kick three times.
3. All kicks are measured at right angles to the kicking line.

Scoring

The score is the distance in full feet measured to the last foot passed, disregarding inches, from the kicking line to the point where the longest kick hits the ground.

Dodging Run

Purpose

To measure how fast a player can run and dodge while carrying a football.

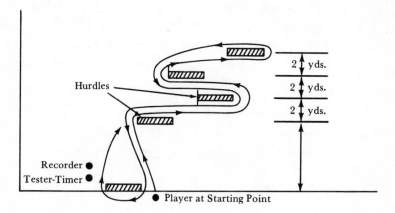

Figure 2.45.

Equipment

A football field or other smooth grass field, standard footballs, five low hurdles, stop watch, measuring tape, line marker.

Description

This test is the Frederick W. Cozens Dodging Test, except that a football is carried. A course is laid out from a starting line on which the first hurdle is placed. The other hurdles are arranged as shown in the diagram. The player stands behind the starting line at the right of the first hurdle with a football in his hands. On the signal "go" he runs around the hurdles and returns as shown in the diagram. He then continues without stopping for a second round trip. Two round trips constitute a run.

Rules

1. The player must warm up before being tested and is allowed one practice run.
2. The ball can be carried in any way and need not be changed from side to side.
3. If the ball is dropped the run does not count.
4. Each player is timed on two runs.

Scoring

The score is the best time in seconds and tenths of seconds required to make two round trips over the course, timed from the signal "go" until the instant the player crosses the starting line at the end of the second round trip. The better of the two times is the player's score.

FORWARD PASS FOR DISTANCE

Percentile Scores Based on Age / Test Scores in Feet

Percentile	AGE								Percentile
	10	11	12	13	14	15	16	17-18	
100th	96	105	120	150	170	180	180	180	100th
95th	71	83	99	115	126	135	144	152	95th
90th	68	76	92	104	118	127	135	143	90th
85th	64	73	87	98	114	122	129	137	85th
80th	62	70	83	95	109	118	126	133	80th
75th	61	68	79	91	105	115	123	129	75th
70th	59	65	77	88	102	111	120	127	70th
65th	58	64	75	85	99	108	117	124	65th
60th	56	62	73	83	96	105	114	121	60th
55th	55	61	71	80	93	102	111	117	55th
50th	53	59	68	78	91	99	108	114	50th
45th	52	56	66	76	88	97	105	110	45th
40th	51	54	64	73	85	94	103	107	40th
35th	49	51	62	70	83	92	100	104	35th
30th	47	50	60	69	80	89	97	101	30th
25th	45	48	58	65	77	85	93	98	25th
20th	44	45	54	63	73	81	90	94	20th
15th	41	43	51	61	70	76	85	89	15th
10th	38	40	45	55	64	71	79	80	10th
5th	33	36	40	46	53	62	70	67	5th
0	14	25	10	10	10	20	30	20	0

50-YARD DASH WITH FOOTBALL

Table 2.39

Percentile Scores Based on Age / Test Scores in Seconds and Tenths

Percentile	AGE								Percentile
	10	11	12	13	14	15	16	17-18	
100th	7.3	6.8	6.2	5.5	5.5	5.5	5.5	5.0	100th
95th	7.7	7.4	7.0	6.5	6.5	6.2	6.0	6.0	95th
90th	7.9	7.6	7.2	6.8	6.6	6.3	6.1	6.1	90th
85th	8.1	7.7	7.4	6.9	6.8	6.4	6.3	6.2	85th
80th	8.2	7.8	7.5	7.0	6.9	6.5	6.4	6.3	80th
75th	8.3	7.9	7.5	7.1	7.0	6.6	6.5	6.3	75th
70th	8.4	8.0	7.6	7.2	7.1	6.7	6.6	6.4	70th
65th	8.5	8.1	7.7	7.3	7.2	6.8	6.6	6.5	65th
60th	8.6	8.2	7.8	7.4	7.2	6.9	6.7	6.6	60th
55th	8.6	8.3	7.9	7.5	7.3	7.0	6.8	6.6	55th
50th	8.7	8.4	8.0	7.5	7.4	7.0	6.8	6.7	50th
45th	8.8	8.5	8.1	7.6	7.5	7.1	6.9	6.8	45th
40th	8.9	8.6	8.1	7.7	7.6	7.2	7.0	6.8	40th
35th	9.0	8.7	8.2	7.8	7.7	7.2	7.1	6.9	35th
30th	9.1	8.8	8.3	8.0	7.8	7.3	7.2	7.0	30th
25th	9.2	8.9	8.4	8.1	7.9	7.4	7.3	7.1	25th
20th	9.3	9.1	8.5	8.2	8.1	7.5	7.4	7.2	20th
15th	9.4	9.2	8.7	8.4	8.3	7.7	7.5	7.3	15th
10th	9.6	9.3	9.0	8.7	8.4	8.1	7.8	7.4	10th
5th	9.8	9.5	9.3	9.0	8.8	8.4	8.0	7.8	5th
0	10.6	11.0	12.0	12.0	12.0	11.0	10.0	10.0	0

127

Table 2.40

BLOCKING

Percentile Scores Based on Age / Test Scores in Seconds and Tenths

Percentile	10	11	12	13	14	15	16	17-18	Percentile
100th	6.9	5.0	5.0	5.0	5.0	5.0	5.0	5.0	100th
95th	7.5	6.6	6.6	5.9	5.8	5.8	5.8	5.5	95th
90th	7.7	7.1	7.1	6.5	6.2	6.2	6.1	5.7	90th
85th	7.9	7.5	7.5	6.7	6.6	6.3	6.3	5.8	85th
80th	8.1	8.0	7.7	6.9	6.8	6.5	6.5	6.0	80th
75th	8.3	8.3	7.9	7.2	7.0	6.7	6.7	6.2	75th
70th	8.5	8.6	8.1	7.4	7.1	6.9	7.0	6.3	70th
65th	8.9	9.1	8.4	7.6	7.3	7.0	7.2	6.5	65th
60th	9.3	9.5	8.6	7.7	7.5	7.2	7.4	6.7	60th
55th	9.6	9.7	8.8	7.9	7.7	7.4	7.6	7.0	55th
50th	9.8	9.9	9.0	8.1	7.8	7.5	7.8	7.2	50th
45th	10.1	10.2	9.2	8.3	8.0	7.8	8.0	7.4	45th
40th	10.5	10.4	9.4	8.4	8.1	7.9	8.3	7.6	40th
35th	10.7	10.6	9.6	8.6	8.3	8.2	8.6	7.8	35th
30th	11.0	10.9	9.7	8.9	8.5	8.3	8.8	8.0	30th
25th	11.3	11.1	9.9	9.1	8.7	8.5	9.1	8.2	25th
20th	11.6	11.3	10.2	9.4	9.0	8.8	9.5	8.5	20th
15th	12.0	11.6	10.5	9.8	9.2	9.0	9.0	8.9	15th
10th	12.8	12.0	10.9	10.2	9.5	9.4	10.6	9.4	10th
5th	14.4	13.1	11.6	11.2	10.3	10.4	10.7	10.8	5th
0	17.5	18.0	15.0	15.0	15.0	13.0	15.0	14.0	0

FORWARD PASS FOR ACCURACY

Percentile Scores Based on Age / Test Scores in Points

Percentile	10	11	12	13	14	15	16	17-18	Percentile
100th	18	26	26	26	26	26	28	28	100th
95th	14	19	20	21	21	21	21	22	95th
90th	11	16	18	19	19	19	20	21	90th
85th	10	15	17	18	18	18	18	19	85th
80th	9	13	16	17	17	17	17	18	80th
75th	8	12	15	16	16	16	16	18	75th
70th	8	11	14	15	15	15	15	17	70th
65th	6	10	13	14	14	14	15	16	65th
60th	5	9	12	13	13	13	14	15	60th
55th	4	8	11	13	13	13	13	15	55th
50th	3	7	11	12	12	12	13	14	50th
45th	2	6	10	11	11	11	12	13	45th
40th	2	5	9	11	10	11	12	12	40th
35th	1	5	8	10	9	9	11	12	35th
30th	0	4	7	9	8	9	10	11	30th
25th	0	3	6	8	8	8	9	10	25th
20th	0	2	5	7	7	7	8	9	20th
15th	0	1	4	5	5	6	7	8	15th
10th	0	0	3	4	4	5	6	7	10th
5th	0	0	1	2	2	3	4	5	5th
0	0	0	0	0	0	0	0	0	0

Table 2.41

FOOTBALL PUNT FOR DISTANCE

Percentile Scores Based on Age / Test Scores in Feet

Percentile	10	11	12	13	14	15	16	17-18	Percentile
100th	87	100	115	150	160	160	160	180	100th
95th	75	84	93	106	119	126	131	136	95th
90th	64	77	88	98	110	119	126	128	90th
85th	61	75	84	94	106	114	120	124	85th
80th	58	70	79	90	103	109	114	120	80th
75th	56	68	77	87	98	105	109	115	75th
70th	55	66	75	83	96	102	106	110	70th
65th	53	64	72	80	93	99	103	107	65th
60th	51	62	70	78	90	96	100	104	60th
55th	50	60	68	75	87	94	97	101	55th
50th	48	57	66	73	84	91	95	98	50th
45th	46	55	64	70	81	89	92	96	45th
40th	45	53	61	68	78	86	90	93	40th
35th	44	51	59	64	75	83	86	90	35th
30th	42	48	56	63	72	79	83	86	30th
25th	40	45	52	61	70	76	79	81	25th
20th	38	42	50	57	66	73	74	76	20th
15th	32	39	46	52	61	69	70	70	15th
10th	28	34	40	44	55	62	64	64	10th
5th	22	27	35	33	44	54	56	53	5th
0	11	9	10	10	10	10	10	10	0

BALL CHANGING ZIGZAG RUN

Percentile Scores Based on Age / Test Scores in Seconds and Tenths

Percentile	10	11	12	13	14	15	16	17-18	Percentile
100th	7.2	7.4	7.0	6.0	6.5	6.0	6.0	6.0	100th
95th	9.9	7.7	7.8	8.0	8.7	7.7	7.7	8.4	95th
90th	10.1	8.1	8.2	8.4	9.0	8.0	8.0	8.7	90th
85th	10.3	8.6	8.5	8.7	9.2	8.3	8.4	8.8	85th
80th	10.5	9.0	8.7	8.8	9.4	8.5	8.6	8.9	80th
75th	10.7	9.3	8.8	9.0	9.5	8.6	8.7	9.0	75th
70th	10.9	9.6	9.0	9.2	9.6	8.7	8.8	9.1	70th
65th	11.1	9.8	9.1	9.3	9.7	8.8	8.9	9.2	65th
60th	11.2	10.0	9.3	9.5	9.8	8.9	9.0	9.3	60th
55th	11.4	10.1	9.5	9.6	9.9	9.0	9.1	9.4	55th
50th	11.5	10.3	9.6	9.7	10.0	9.1	9.3	9.6	50th
45th	11.6	10.5	9.8	9.8	10.1	9.2	9.4	9.7	45th
40th	11.8	10.6	10.0	10.0	10.2	9.4	9.5	9.8	40th
35th	11.9	10.9	10.1	10.2	10.4	9.5	9.7	9.9	35th
30th	12.2	11.1	10.3	10.3	10.5	9.6	9.9	10.1	30th
25th	12.5	11.3	10.5	10.3	10.7	9.9	10.1	10.3	25th
20th	12.8	11.6	10.8	10.8	10.9	10.1	10.3	10.5	20th
15th	13.3	12.1	11.1	11.1	11.2	10.3	10.6	10.9	15th
10th	13.8	12.9	11.5	11.4	11.5	10.6	11.2	11.4	10th
5th	15.8	14.2	12.3	12.1	12.0	11.5	12.2	12.1	5th
0	24.0	15.0	19.0	20.0	14.5	20.0	17.0	15.0	0

Table 2.42

CATCHING THE FORWARD PASS

Percentile Scores Based on Age / Test Scores in Number Caught

Percentile	AGE								Percentile
	10	11	12	13	14	15	16	17-18	
100th	20	20	20	20	20	20	20	20	100th
95th	19	19	19	20	20	20	20	20	95th
90th	17	18	19	19	19	19	19	19	90th
85th	16	16	18	18	18	19	19	19	85th
80th	14	15	18	17	18	18	18	18	80th
75th	13	14	16	17	17	18	18	18	75th
70th	12	13	16	16	16	17	17	17	70th
65th	11	12	15	15	15	16	16	16	65th
60th	10	12	14	15	15	16	16	16	60th
55th	8	11	14	14	14	15	15	15	55th
50th	7	10	13	13	14	15	15	15	50th
45th	7	9	12	13	13	14	14	14	45th
40th	6	8	12	12	12	13	13	13	40th
35th	5	7	11	11	11	12	12	13	35th
30th	5	7	10	10	10	11	11	12	30th
25th	4	6	10	9	9	10	10	11	25th
20th	3	5	8	8	8	9	9	10	20th
15th	2	4	7	7	8	8	8	9	15th
10th	1	3	6	6	6	7	6	8	10th
5th	1	1	5	4	4	6	4	6	5th
0	0	0	0	0	0	0	0	0	0

PULL-OUT

Percentile Scores Based on Age / Test Scores in Seconds and Tenths

Percentile	AGE								Percentile
	10	11	12	13	14	15	16	17-18	
100th	2.5	2.2	2.2	2.2	2.2	2.0	2.0	1.8	100th
95th	2.9	2.8	2.8	2.8	2.7	2.5	2.5	2.5	95th
90th	3.2	3.0	3.0	2.9	2.8	2.6	2.6	2.6	90th
85th	3.3	3.0	3.0	3.0	2.9	2.7	2.7	2.7	85th
80th	3.4	3.1	3.1	3.0	3.0	2.8	2.9	2.8	80th
75th	3.5	3.1	3.1	3.1	3.0	3.0	2.9	2.9	75th
70th	3.5	3.2	3.2	3.1	3.0	3.0	3.0	2.9	70th
65th	3.6	3.3	3.3	3.2	3.1	3.0	3.0	3.0	65th
60th	3.6	3.3	3.3	3.2	3.1	3.1	3.1	3.0	60th
55th	3.7	3.3	3.3	3.3	3.2	3.1	3.1	3.1	55th
50th	3.8	3.4	3.4	3.3	3.2	3.2	3.2	3.1	50th
45th	3.8	3.5	3.5	3.4	3.3	3.2	3.2	3.1	45th
40th	3.9	3.6	3.5	3.4	3.3	3.3	3.3	3.2	40th
35th	3.9	3.7	3.6	3.5	3.4	3.3	3.3	3.2	35th
30th	4.0	3.8	3.7	3.5	3.4	3.4	3.3	3.2	30th
25th	4.0	3.9	3.8	3.6	3.5	3.5	3.4	3.3	25th
20th	4.1	4.0	3.9	3.7	3.5	3.6	3.5	3.4	20th
15th	4.2	4.1	3.9	3.8	3.6	3.7	3.7	3.5	15th
10th	4.3	4.2	4.1	3.9	3.7	3.9	3.9	3.6	10th
5th	4.4	4.4	4.2	4.0	4.0	4.1	4.3	3.9	5th
0	5.5	5.0	5.0	5.0	5.0	5.0	5.0	5.0	0

Table 2.43

KICK-OFF

Percentile Scores Based on Age / Test Scores in Feet

Percentile	AGE								Percentile
	10	11	12	13	14	15	16	17-18	
100th	88	110	120	129	140	160	160	180	100th
95th	69	79	98	106	118	128	131	138	95th
90th	64	72	83	97	108	120	125	129	90th
85th	59	68	78	92	102	114	119	124	85th
80th	58	64	74	86	97	108	114	119	80th
75th	55	60	70	81	94	104	108	113	75th
70th	53	58	67	78	90	100	104	108	70th
65th	50	56	65	75	86	96	99	105	65th
60th	47	54	64	72	84	93	97	103	60th
55th	46	52	60	69	81	90	95	98	55th
50th	45	50	57	67	77	87	93	95	50th
45th	43	48	54	64	74	83	90	92	45th
40th	40	46	52	62	71	79	87	88	40th
35th	39	44	48	59	68	76	83	84	35th
30th	37	42	45	56	65	72	79	79	30th
25th	35	40	42	52	62	69	75	74	25th
20th	32	37	38	48	58	64	70	70	20th
15th	30	34	34	42	52	59	65	64	15th
10th	26	30	29	36	45	50	60	57	10th
5th	21	24	22	26	38	40	47	43	5th
0	5	10	0	0	0	10	10	10	0

DODGING RUN

Percentile Scores Based on Age / Test Scores in Seconds and Tenths

Percentile	AGE								Percentile
	10	11	12	13	14	15	16	17-18	
100th	21.0	18.0	18.0	17.0	16.0	16.0	16.0	16.0	100th
95th	24.3	23.8	23.8	23.3	22.6	22.4	22.3	22.2	95th
90th	25.8	24.6	24.6	24.2	23.9	23.5	23.3	23.2	90th
85th	26.3	25.0	25.0	24.8	24.6	24.1	23.9	23.7	85th
80th	26.4	25.2	25.2	24.9	24.7	24.6	24.3	24.1	80th
75th	27.5	25.3	25.3	25.3	25.2	24.9	24.7	24.4	75th
70th	27.8	25.8	25.8	25.7	25.2	25.2	25.0	24.7	70th
65th	28.1	26.3	26.3	26.1	26.1	25.5	25.3	25.0	65th
60th	28.4	26.6	26.6	26.5	26.3	25.8	25.5	25.3	60th
55th	28.7	26.9	26.9	26.8	26.6	26.1	25.8	25.6	55th
50th	28.9	27.4	27.3	27.2	26.9	26.4	26.1	26.0	50th
45th	29.3	28.0	27.6	27.5	27.2	26.7	26.3	26.3	45th
40th	29.7	28.3	27.9	27.9	27.5	27.0	26.7	26.6	40th
35th	30.1	28.8	28.4	28.3	27.9	27.4	27.0	26.9	35th
30th	30.5	29.2	28.8	28.7	28.3	27.8	27.3	27.2	30th
25th	30.9	29.8	29.2	29.1	28.7	28.2	27.7	27.6	25th
20th	31.3	30.4	29.8	29.5	29.3	28.6	28.1	28.0	20th
15th	31.8	31.1	30.4	30.1	29.9	29.1	28.8	28.7	15th
10th	32.7	32.0	31.3	30.8	30.7	29.8	29.6	29.2	10th
5th	33.6	33.5	33.0	32.3	31.8	31.0	30.6	30.4	5th
0	40.0	40.0	41.0	40.0	36.0	36.0	36.0	36.0	0

GOLF SKILL TESTS*
INSTRUCTIONS FOR ADMINISTERING TESTS

Chip Test

Purpose

To measure the ability of the student to control a golf ball on a chip or pitch and run shot.

Test Area

An athletic field with three trapezoids marked on the ground with measurements as shown in Figure 2.46. A shooting line is located 18 feet from the front of the center target.

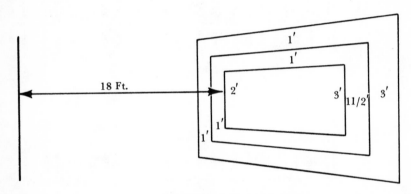

Figure 2.46. Target For Chip Test.

Shots

A test consists of 15 shots.

Scoring

The balls are scored on the basis of the point that they first strike the ground with 3, 2, and 1 points for the inner, middle, and outer trapezoids respectively. Whiffs and shots that fail to strike in the target area are scored zero. Balls striking a line are given the score of the highest adjacent area.

*H. Steven Brown, "A Test Battery for Evaluating Golf Skills." *TAHPER Journal,* May 1969, Pages 4-5, 28-29. Used by permission of the author.

Short Pitch Test

Purpose

To measure the ability of the student to hit the desired target area on a pitch shot.

Test Area

An athletic field with three concentric circles marked on the ground as shown in Figure 2.47 and with radii of 7 1/2, 15, and 22 1/2 feet for the center, middle, and outer circles respectively. The shooting arc is located 65 feet from the center of the inner circle.

Shots

A trial consists of 15 shots.

Scoring

The balls are scored on the basis of the point that they first strike the ground with 3, 2, and 1 respectively for the inner, middle, and outer circles. Whiffs and shots that fail to strike the target area are scored zero.

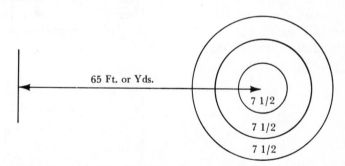

Figure 2.47. Target For Short Pitch Test and Approach Test.

Approach Test

Purpose

To measure the ability of the student to stop the golf ball at a desired point.

Test Area

An athletic field or golf course with three concentric circles marked on the ground as in Figure 2.47 but with radii of 7 1/2, 15, and 22 1/2 yards rather than feet. The shooting arc is located 65 yards from the center of the target area.

Shots

A trial consists of 15 shots.

Scoring

The scoring is identical to that used for the Short Pitch Test except that the score is based on where the ball stops and comes to rest rather than where it first hits.

Driving Test

Purpose

To measure the ability of the student to drive a golf ball accurately and for distance.

Test Area

An athletic field or golf course with two lines of markers located 50 yards apart with markers in each line being located every 50 yards as shown in Figure 2.48. Two tees are located at the end of the range and between the lines of targets.

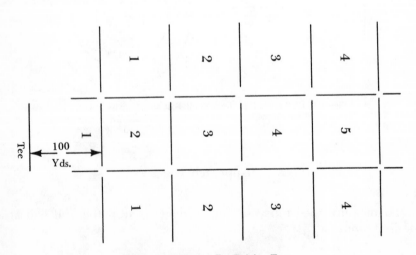

Figure 2.48. Target For Driving Test.

Shots

The test consists of 9 shots.

Scoring

Balls are scored on the basis of the area in which they come to rest and are given points as indicated in Figure 2.48.

Putting Test

Purpose

To measure the putting ability of the student.

Test Area

The test area is a slightly rolling putting green with six holes, two about 15 feet and four about 20 feet long. One hole is downhill and one uphill; one breaks to the left and one to the right, and two are on a level surface. Each school will have to develop local norms for this test.

Procedure

The students are tested in pairs moving around the course in a clockwise direction. Each student puts 12 holes, sinking all shots; none are conceded.

Scoring

The total number of strokes needed to put 12 holes is converted to a point score by the norms below so that it may be compared with the scores of the other tests.

Strokes	Score	Strokes	Score	Strokes	Score
21	45	29	29	37	13
22	43	30	27	38	11
23	41	31	25	39	9
24	39	32	23	40	7
25	37	33	21	41	5
26	35	34	19	42	3
27	33	35	17	43	1
28	31	36	15	44	0

Table 2.44

T-Scales for Brown's Revised Golf Skill Test

Raw Score	Chip Men	Chip Women	Pitch Men	Pitch Women	Approach Men	Approach Women	Driving Men	Driving Women	Putting Men	Putting Women
45	71	87	69	89	72	84	71	-- --	72	75
44	70	86	68	88	70	83	70	100	71	74
43	69	85	67	86	69	81	68	99	69	73
42	67	83	66	85	68	80	67	97	68	71
41	66	82	64	84	67	79	66	95	66	70
40	65	81	63	82	66	77	65	93	65	69
39	64	80	62	81	64	76	64	92	64	68
38	63	78	61	80	63	75	62	90	62	67
37	62	77	60	78	62	73	61	88	61	66
36	60	76	59	77	61	72	60	86	59	65
35	59	74	58	76	59	71	59	84	58	63
34	58	73	56	75	58	69	57	82	56	62
33	57	72	55	73	58	68	56	80	55	61
32	56	70	54	72	56	67	55	78	53	60
31	55	69	53	71	56	66	54	76	52	59
30	54	68	52	69	54	64	53	75	51	58
29	52	66	51	68	53	63	51	73	49	57
28	51	65	50	67	52	61	50	71	48	55
27	50	64	48	65	50	60	49	69	46	54
26	49	62	47	64	49	59	48	67	45	53
25	48	61	46	63	48	58	46	65	43	52
24	47	60	45	62	47	56	45	63	42	51
23	45	59	44	60	45	55	44	62	40	50
22	44	57	43	59	44	54	43	60	39	49
21	43	56	42	58	43	52	42	58	38	47
20	42	55	40	56	42	51	40	56	36	46
19	41	53	39	55	41	50	39	54	35	45
18	40	52	38	54	40	49	38	52	33	44
17	38	51	37	52	38	47	37	50	32	43
16	37	49	36	51	37	46	35	48	30	42
15	36	48	35	50	36	44	34	46	29	40
14	35	47	33	49	35	43	33	44	27	39
13	34	46	32	47	34	42	32	43	26	38
12	33	44	31	46	32	40	31	41	25	37
11	31	43	30	45	31	39	29	39	23	36
10	30	42	29	43	30	38	28	37	22	35
9	29	40	28	42	29	36	27	35	20	34
8	28	39	27	41	28	35	26	33	21	32
7	27	38	25	39	27	34	25	31	19	31
6	26	36	24	38	25	32	23	30	18	30
5	24	35	23	37	24	31	22	28	16	29
4	23	34	22	36	23	30	21	26	15	28
3	22	32	21	34	21	29	20	24	14	27
2	21	31	20	33	20	28	18	22	12	26
1	20	30	19	32	19	27	17	20	11	24
Number	518	514	599	508	561	531	253	192	458	436

SOCCER SKILL TEST*

Purpose

To measure present skills in soccer and to provide a classification and playing ability status.

Sex and Age Level

High school boys and girls, college men and women, and varsity players.

Test Items and Equipment

Obstacle Run

An area 44 yards long and approximately 20 yards wide, one stop watch, one regulation soccer goal, individual scorecards, and one soccer ball (three preferable) are needed.

Accuracy Kick

Two lines six yards long run parallel to the goal line, one 11 yards and one 12 yards from the goal line. Eight chalked lines are marked perpendicular to the goal line; one on either side of the goal post, one drawn from each of the goal posts, and four marked between the goal posts. These division lines should be three yards long and three feet six inches apart. It is suggested that ropes or cords be tied to the crossbar, stretched to the ground, and fastened with pegs along the goal line at the designated scoring areas. The scoring for the accuracy-kick areas should be chalked on the ground in 1·3·2·1·2·3·1 order (see figure) with the highest point value nearest the goal posts and the lowest value in the center scoring area. Additional markings may be used to facilitate accuracy in scoring by using oil cloth squares with the point value of each division marked on them. These squares should be attached to the crossbar and hung between each of the divisions. The same soccer ball is used throughout the test.

Leadership

Obstacle Run

One person acts as the starter (rolls ball to subject for attempted trap). One person is located at the six-yard accuracy-kick line to

---

*Tomlinson, Rebecca, "Soccer Skill Test," *Soccer-Speedball Guide,* 1964-1966. Division of Girls' and Women's Sports, American Association for Health, Physical Education, and Recreation. Used by permission of the AAHPER.

indicate to the timer the moment the ball is kicked by the subject (lowering or raising the arm may be used as the signal) and to record both phases of the test. Four people (class members) are to be stationed as obstacles at the four designated spots on the obstacle course.

Accuracy Kick

One person (a student may be used) indicates the point value of the accuracy kick. There are two ball chasers (students).

Time Requirements and Number That Can Be Tested

Approximately 45 subjects may complete the test (one trial) during a 50 minute period. It is suggested that two testing stations be used if goal posts and necessary areas are available, one station on each half of the playing field.

Space Planning

This test may be organized on a regular soccer field. If a regular field is not available, an area 44 yards long and approximately 20 feet wide with regulation goal posts may be used. See figure 2.49 for the suggested layout for the testing.

Demonstration of Test

It is suggested that the skills used during the test, trapping, dribbling, and kicking be demonstrated prior to the actual testing. The entire test should be demonstrated for the subjects to be tested.

Instructions To Be Read To Subjects

The purpose of these tests is to measure your ability to trap, your speed and agility in dribbling, and your accuracy in kicking a soccer ball. As you get in position to begin your test the leader will indicate to you whether you are to aim at the right or the left of the scoring area when attempting your accuracy kick. Stand behind the starting line. The leader will roll the ball to you, and the instant the ball reaches the starting line you are to trap the ball and start your dribble around the obstacle course. *The ball must be in a stationary position behind the starting line before you may start your obstacle path even though time will be recorded the instant you make contact with the ball.* If you should lose control of the ball while dribbling, regain control and continue following the correct path of the course. You are to continue dribbling as fast as you can until you reach the accuracy-kick line. Upon crossing the accuracy-kick line and before you reach the chalked line one yard parallel to the kick line, attempt to kick the ball between the goal posts, under the crossbar, and toward the direction indicated to you prior to the starting of your test (either to the right or left of the center of the scoring area).

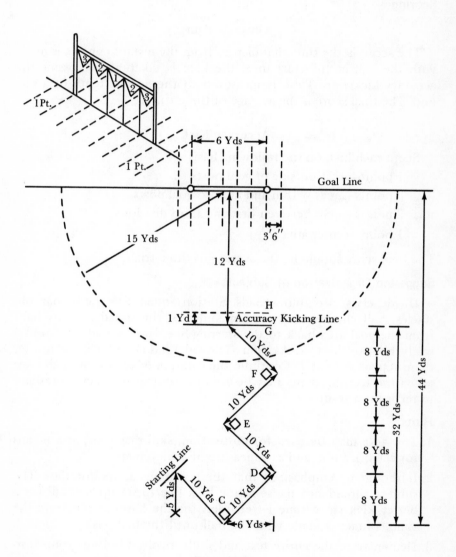

Figure 2.49.

Your time score is recorded from the time you first make contact with the ball on the starting line until you have crossed the accuracy-kick line. Your accuracy score is determined by the point area through which the ball passes at the goal line.

Scoring

Obstacle Run

The score is the time that elapses from the instant contact is made with the ball at the start until the kick is taken after crossing the accuracy-kick line. Time is measured to the nearest tenth of a second. The final score is the average of three trials.

Accuracy Kick

Score each kick on the following basis:

1 point—areas outside of goal posts

3 points—areas within and next to goal posts

2 points—areas between first and third divisions

1 point—center area

The final score should be the average of three trials.

Suggested Organization of Subjects

Divide class into four squads. Station Squad 4 as the human obstacles, ball chasers, and the remainder of the squad to relay balls from the goal area back to the starting line. Have Squads 1, 2, and 3 ready to take the test. As soon as Squad 1 has completed the test let them replace Squad 4. Continue the rotation of squads until all have taken the test. Students may be used to confirm accuracy scores and to record test results.

Hints

1. This test may be used for motivation, skill diagnosis, as a means for classification, and as a measure of achievement.

2. It should be emphasized that the test items are continuous. The subject should not pause at the kick line to set up the ball for a better kick since time is recorded for the obstacle run from the time contact is made with the ball until the ball has been kicked.

3. Demonstrate the entire test and skills involved before group testing.

SOFTBALL SKILL TESTS*

Throw For Distance

Purpose

To measure distance a softball can be thrown.

Equipment

A smooth grass or dirt field with throwing zone lines marked and, preferably, five-yard lines marked, softballs, measuring tape, stake markers.

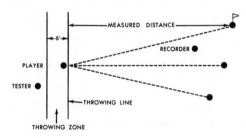

Figure 2.50.

Description

A throwing line is marked off at one end of the field and a line parallel to and six feet from it is also marked, thus forming a zone 6 feet wide from which the throw is to be made. The player takes position in the throwing zone with a softball in hand, takes one or two steps and throws as far as possible and as nearly at right angles to the throwing line as possible. He may throw with either hand. A small marking stake is placed at the point at which the ball first hits the ground. If the second or third throw is farther the stake is moved to the new point. (It speeds up measuring if the player goes out and stands by his stake; after four or five players have thrown, all their distances can be measured at the same time.) Players must be

---

*AAHPER, *Softball Skills Test Manual for Boys* and *Softball Skills Test Manual for Girls,* Washington, D.C. American Association for Health, Physical Education, and Recreation, (1201 16th St. N.W., Washington, D.C.). Used by permission of the AAHPER.

warmed up before throwing. (This test is the same as the softball throw in the *AAHPER Youth Fitness Test Manual.*)

Rules

1. Throws must be made from within the throwing zone.
2. One or more running steps may be taken in making the throw.
3. Throws must be measured at right angles to the throwing line.
4. Three throws are allowed.

Scoring

The score is the distance of the farthest throw. The distance from the throwing line to the stake for the farthest throw is measured at right angles to the throwing line. Throws are measured to the nearest foot. Record the distance of the best throw on the squad score card.

Overhand Throw For Accuracy

Purpose

To measure accuracy with which a softball can be thrown from a distance about that required for an infielder's throw to a base or home plate.

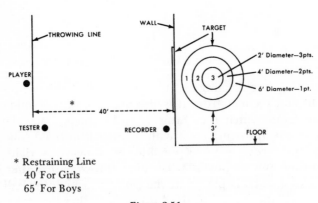

* Restraining Line
40' For Girls
65' For Boys

Figure 2.51.

Equipment

A gymnasium or outdoor space adjacent to a smooth wall on which the target can be placed, a target (see diagram) painted on canvas or marked on the wall, softballs, measuring tape, chalk.

Description

The target consists of three concentric circles marked by lines one inch wide painted on a sheet of canvas at least 8 feet square, or painted or marked with chalk on a smooth wall, or on a large mat hung on a wall. The center circle is 2 feet in diameter (outside measurement), the next circle 4 feet in diameter, and the outer circle 6 feet in diameter. The bottom of the outer circle is exactly 3 feet above the floor. The throw is made from behind a line parallel to and 40 feet from the face of the target. After one or two practice throws, the player takes ten throws.

Rules

1. Throws must be made with both feet behind the throwing line.
2. One or two steps can be taken in making the throw.
3. Ten throws are taken.

Scoring

Balls hitting in the center circle count 3 points, balls hitting in the next area count 2 points, and balls hitting in the outer area count 1 point. Balls hitting on a line count as the higher number of points. The score is the sum of points made on ten throws. Record points on each throw as made. The maximum score is 30 points.

Underhand Pitching

Purpose

To measure accuracy with which a softball can be pitched.

Equipment

A gymnasium or outdoor space adjacent to a smooth wall, a target as shown in the diagram, softballs, measuring tape, chalk.

Description

The target is rectangular with an inner rectangle 17 inches wide and 30 inches high and an outer rectangle which is 6 inches larger on all sides. Lines (one-inch wide) are painted on canvas or marked on a wall. The target is placed so that the bottom of the outer rectangle is exactly 18 inches above the floor. A pitching line 24 inches long is marked on the floor opposite the center of the target and parallel to the face of the target. This line is 38 feet from the target. The player is allowed one practice pitch and then takes 15 underhand pitches at the target. The player must keep one foot on the pitching line while delivering the ball but can take a forward step in making the pitch.

Rules

1. A legal underhand softball pitch must be used.
2. One foot must be in contact with the pitching line until the ball has been delivered.
3. Fifteen pitches are taken.

Scoring

Pitched balls hitting in the center area or on its boundary line count 2 points, and balls hitting in the outer area or on its outside boundary line count 1 point. The score is the sum of all points made on 15 pitches. Record each score as made. The maximum score is 30 points.

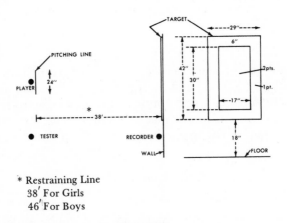

* Restraining Line
38' For Girls
46' For Boys

Figure 2.52.

SPEED THROW

Purpose

To measure speed with which a player can handle the ball in catching and throwing.

Equipment

A gymnasium with a smooth wall or outside area with a smooth ground surface and a smooth wall, softballs, stop watch.

Description

A line is drawn on the floor parallel to and 9 feet from a solid smooth wall with a clear space of 8 to 10 feet in width and height.

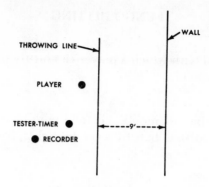

Figure 2.53.

The player stands behind the line with a softball in hand. She throws the ball overhead against the wall and catches the rebound, and continues throwing and catching as rapidly as possible until she has completed 15 hits on the wall. Balls must be thrown overhand and should hit the wall about head high or a bit higher for best results. Players start on signal "go" but time is started when the ball hits the wall. Balls which fall short can be retrieved, but the player must return and throw from behind the line. Two trials are timed. A practice trial is allowed.

Rules

1. Any method of catching may be used but overhand one-hand throws must be made.
2. Bad bounces or dropped balls can be retrieved but the player must return to behind the line before resuming throwing and catching.
3. If the ball gets entirely away, one new trial may be given.
4. Two trials are given.

Scoring

The score is the time in seconds and tenths of seconds required for the 15 consecutive hits on the wall, timed from the instant the first ball hits the wall to the instant the fifteenth throw hits the wall. Both times are recorded on the squad score card. The time on the best of two trials is the player's score.

FUNGO HITTING

Purpose

To measure skill with which a player can hit fly balls alternately to right field and left field.

Equipment

A standard softball diamond and field with base lines marked and bases in position, softball bats of several weights, softballs.

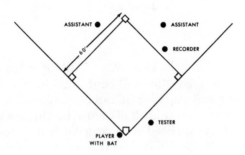

Figure 2.54.

Description

The player stands behind home plate with a bat of her choice and a ball in hand. She tosses the ball up and tries to hit a fly ball into right field. She then tries to hit the next fly ball into left field. She continues hitting to the right and left alternately until she has tried to hit ten balls to each side. A ball missed entirely does not count as a trial unless two balls are missed in succession. Each time the bat touches a ball it counts as a trial regardless of where the ball goes. After each hit the player's next hit must be aimed at the opposite side. The tester can call "right" or "left" to indicate the side to which the next hit is to go. Hits intended for a specific side must cross the base line between second and third base or first and second base. Practice trials to each side are allowed. Assistants may retrieve balls.

Rules

1. The player must try to hit to alternate sides.

2. Two entirely missed balls in succession count as a trial.

3. Twenty hits are taken (ten to each direction).

Scoring

The score is the sum of points made on twenty hits, taken alternately to right and left for ten hits to each side. Fly balls which land beyond the base line on the intended side count 2 points, while ground balls hit across the base line on the intended side count 1 point. When hits intended for right field land at the left of second base no score is made, and similarly when balls intended for left field go to the right of second base no score is made. Record each point as made. The maximum score is 40 points.

BASE RUNNING

Purpose

To measure the speed with which a player can run around the bases after a swing at an imaginary pitch.

Equipment

A standard softball field and diamond with home plate, bases, and a batter's box laid out for a right-handed batter; softball bats; stop watch.

Description

The player takes her position in the right-hand batter's box, holding a bat as if ready for a pitch. On the signal "hit" the player swings at an imaginary ball, drops the bat (it must not be thrown), and runs around the bases being careful to touch each base. A practice run is allowed. Two trials are taken.

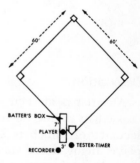

Figure 2.55.

Rules

1. The player must stand in the batter's box for a right-handed batter.

2. The player must complete her swing with the bat before starting to run.

3. The bat must be dropped, not thrown or carried.

4. The player must touch each base in turn on the run.

5. Two runs are taken.

Scoring

Trials are timed in seconds and tenths of seconds from the signal "hit" to the instant the runner touches home plate after circling the bases. Both times are recorded. The best time is the score.

FIELDING GROUND BALLS

Purpose

To measure ability of a player to field ground balls quickly.

Equipment

A smooth area on which markings can be placed, marked off as indicated, softballs, baskets, a sweep-hand watch, measuring tape, marking equipment (lime, tapes, or trenches).

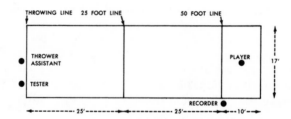

Figure 2.56.

Description

An area is marked out which is 17 feet by 60 feet in size; it is crossed by a line 50 feet from the front or throwing line, and by a second line which is 25 feet from the front or throwing line. The player being tested stands inside the 10-foot area beyond the 50-foot line. An assistant with the basket of ten balls stands back of the throwing line. Spare balls are available to be used if needed. On signal "go" the assistant starts throwing grounders into the marked area at intervals of five seconds. Each throw must strike the ground between the throwing line and the 25-foot line and within the side lines, for at least one bounce. The thrower should throw with good speed, like a machine, with some variation in direction, but not trying to make the fielder miss. The player must field each ball cleanly, hold it momentarily, and toss it aside and be ready for the next ball. The player starts back of the 50-foot line but thereafter fields anywhere back of the 25-foot line. A practice trial is allowed.

Rules

1. The thrower should throw overhand with good speed.
2. The five-second interval between throws must be maintained.
3. Balls must be fielded cleanly inside the prescribed area, held momentarily, and then tossed aside.
4. A throw not made as specified can be taken over. If a series of throws is badly interrupted, it may be repeated at the discretion of the tester.

Scoring

Each ball correctly fielded counts 1 point. Record a point or a zero for each throw. The score is the total of points on 20 throws; the maximum score is 20 points.

CATCHING FLY BALLS (GIRLS)

Purpose

To measure skill in catching fly balls, at frequent intervals, coming from slightly different directions.

Equipment

A standard softball diamond, with boundaries marking a catching zone, as shown in the diagram; softballs; rope and two standards or posts 8 feet high.

Description

The player stands at second base in the center of a 60-foot square. The thrower stands in a restraining zone 5 feet behind home plate and throws fly balls to player as directed. The thrower must throw the ball over the 8-foot high rope, which is fastened between two standards that are located 5 feet in front of home plate. The thrower must throw with regular good speed. Spare balls are available if needed. The player must catch the ball, toss it aside, and be ready immediately to catch the next ball. The tester stands behind the player being tested and indicates to the thrower whether to throw

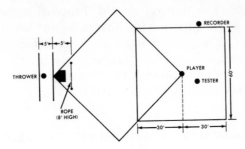

Figure 2.57.

left, right, or straight into the catching zone. Approximately one-third of the balls should be thrown to the right, one-third to the left, and one-third to the middle of the catching zone. Each player is given two trials of ten balls each. A practice trial is allowed.

Rules

1. Balls not thrown properly into the catching zone are not counted.
2. The ball must be thrown so that it describes an arc in flight.
3. A total of 20 good fly balls must be thrown.
4. The player must make a good catch of each ball before tossing it aside.

Scoring

The score is the number of balls successfully caught out of two trials of 10 balls each, for a total of 20 balls. Record one point for each ball caught and zero for misses. (If desired, an X may be recorded for each ball contacted by player but not held.) The maximum score is 20 points.

CATCHING FLYING BALLS (BOYS)

Purpose

To measure skill in catching fly balls, at frequent intervals, coming from slightly different directions.

Equipment

A building of at least two stories high with a window on the second floor which can be opened wide and is 25 to 30 feet above a smooth ground surface (the flat roof of a one-story building can be

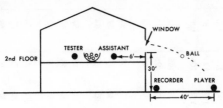

Figure 2.58.

used if the assistant tossing the balls can be out of sight of the player), softballs, baskets.

Description

An assistant takes a position 6 feet from an open second-story window. The player being tested stands on the ground below the window and 30 to 40 feet from the side of the building. On the signal "go" given by the tester the assistant in the building tosses a ball with good speed underhand through the window for the player below to catch. The player must catch the ball, toss it aside, and be ready immediately to catch the next ball. The assistant continues to toss out balls at 10-second intervals until 10 balls have been tossed out. He does not pay any attention as to whether or not the balls are caught. Spare balls are available to be used if needed. The assistant remains entirely out of sight of the player. He should try to vary the direction of the throws slightly but keep the speed constant. The balls are collected in a basket by another assistant and are taken upstairs for use again. The tester or another assistant can help time the throws if desired. If anything happens to interrupt the timing of the throws, the trial can be started over one time. A practice trial is allowed. Two trials of ten throws each are taken.

Rules

1. The player must make a good catch of each ball before tossing it aside.
2. A total of 20 balls must be thrown for catching.

Scoring

The score is the number of balls successfully caught out of two trials of 10 balls each, for a total of 20 balls. Record one point or zero as each ball is caught or missed. The maximum score is 20 points.

Table 2.45

SOFTBALL THROW FOR DISTANCE
Percentile Scores Based on Age / Test Scores in Feet

Percentile	10-11	12	13	14	15	16	17-18	Percentile
100th	200	208	200	230	242	247	255	100th
95th	154	163	185	208	231	229	229	95th
90th	144	152	175	203	205	219	222	90th
85th	127	146	167	191	198	213	216	85th
80th	121	140	160	184	192	208	213	80th
75th	118	135	154	178	187	202	207	75th
70th	114	132	150	173	182	196	204	70th
65th	111	129	145	168	178	193	199	65th
60th	109	125	142	163	174	190	196	60th
55th	106	122	138	159	170	186	192	55th
50th	103	118	135	154	167	183	188	50th
45th	100	115	131	152	165	180	185	45th
40th	98	113	128	148	161	174	182	40th
35th	95	109	125	144	157	171	178	35th
30th	92	106	122	140	154	167	173	30th
25th	91	102	117	137	148	164	169	25th
20th	85	98	113	133	143	159	163	20th
15th	80	93	107	129	138	152	153	15th
10th	72	85	101	123	133	146	147	10th
5th	62	76	97	113	119	140	140	5th
0	24	31	60	105	93	135	90	0

SOFTBALL THROW FOR DISTANCE (GIRLS)
Percentile Scores Based on Age / Test Scores in Feet

Percentile	10-11	12	13	14	15	16	17-18	Percentile
100th	120	160	160	160	200	200	200	100th
95th	99	113	133	126	127	121	120	95th
90th	84	104	112	117	116	109	109	90th
85th	76	98	105	109	108	103	102	85th
80th	71	94	98	104	103	98	97	80th
75th	68	89	94	99	97	94	93	75th
70th	66	85	90	95	93	91	89	70th
65th	62	81	86	92	88	87	87	65th
60th	60	77	83	88	85	84	84	60th
55th	57	74	81	85	80	81	82	55th
50th	55	70	76	82	77	79	80	50th
45th	53	67	73	79	75	76	77	45th
40th	50	64	70	76	72	73	74	40th
35th	48	61	68	73	70	70	72	35th
30th	45	58	64	69	67	67	69	30th
25th	43	55	62	66	64	63	66	25th
20th	41	51	60	61	61	60	63	20th
15th	38	48	56	57	58	56	60	15th
10th	34	43	51	52	54	51	55	10th
5th	31	37	43	43	49	45	50	5th
0	20	20	20	20	20	10	10	0

Table 2.46

OVERHAND THROW FOR ACCURACY
Percentile Scores Based on Age / Test Scores in Points

Percentile	10-11	12	13	AGE 14	15	16	17-18	Percentile
100th	22	22	23	25	25	27	25	100th
95th	14	17	18	19	20	20	21	95th
90th	12	15	16	17	17	18	19	90th
85th	11	13	15	16	16	17	18	85th
80th	9	12	13	15	15	16	17	80th
75th	8	11	12	14	14	15	16	75th
70th	8	11	12	13	13	14	15	70th
65th	7	10	11	12	12	14	15	65th
60th	6	9	10	11	11	13	14	60th
55th	5	9	10	11	11	12	13	55th
50th	5	8	9	10	10	11	13	50th
45th	4	7	8	10	10	11	12	45th
40th	4	6	7	9	9	10	11	40th
35th	3	6	7	8	9	9	11	35th
30th	3	5	6	8	8	8	10	30th
25th	2	4	5	7	7	8	9	25th
20th	1	3	4	6	7	7	8	20th
15th	1	3	3	6	6	6	7	15th
10th	0	2	2	5	5	5	6	10th
5th	0	0	1	3	3	4	4	5th
0	0	0	0	0	0	1	0	0

OVERHAND THROW FOR ACCURACY (GIRLS)
Percentile Scores Based on Age / Test Scores in Points

Percentile	10-11	12	13	AGE 14	15	16	17-18	Percentile
100th	24	26	26	26	30	30	26	100th
95th	17	17	18	19	19	22	20	95th
90th	14	16	16	17	18	20	18	90th
85th	13	14	15	15	16	18	17	85th
80th	12	13	14	14	15	17	16	80th
75th	11	12	13	13	14	16	15	75th
70th	10	11	12	12	13	15	14	70th
65th	9	10	11	11	12	13	13	65th
60th	8	9	10	11	11	12	12	60th
55th	7	9	9	10	11	12	11	55th
50th	6	8	9	9	10	11	10	50th
45th	5	7	8	9	9	10	9	45th
40th	4	6	7	8	8	9	8	40th
35th	4	5	6	7	8	8	7	35th
30th	3	4	6	6	7	7	6	30th
25th	2	4	5	5	6	6	5	25th
20th	1	3	4	4	5	5	4	20th
15th	1	2	3	3	3	4	3	15th
10th	0	1	1	2	2	2	2	10th
5th	0	0	0	1	1	1	1	5th
0	0	0	0	0	0	0	0	0

Table 2.47

UNDERHAND PITCH
Percentile Scores Based on Age / Test Scores in Points

Percentile	10-11	12	13	14	15	16	17-18	Percentile
100th	18	23	21	22	24	25	25	100th
95th	12	14	15	16	18	19	19	95th
90th	10	12	13	15	16	17	17	90th
85th	9	11	11	14	15	15	16	85th
80th	8	9	10	12	14	14	15	80th
75th	7	9	10	12	13	13	14	75th
70th	7	8	9	11	12	12	13	70th
65th	6	7	8	10	11	12	12	65th
60th	6	7	8	9	10	11	12	60th
55th	5	6	7	9	10	10	11	55th
50th	4	6	7	8	9	9	10	50th
45th	4	5	6	7	8	9	10	45th
40th	3	4	5	7	7	8	9	40th
35th	3	4	5	6	7	8	8	35th
30th	2	3	4	6	6	7	8	30th
25th	2	3	4	5	5	6	7	25th
20th	1	2	3	4	4	5	6	20th
15th	1	2	3	4	4	4	5	15th
10th	1	1	2	3	3	3	4	10th
5th	0	0	1	2	2	2	3	5th
0	0	0	0	0	0	0	0	0

UNDERHAND PITCH (GIRLS)
Percentile Scores Based on Age / Test Scores in Points

Percentile	10-11	12	13	14	15	16	17-18	Percentile
100th	23	22	24	24	26	27	26	100th
95th	12	14	16	17	16	19	21	95th
90th	10	13	14	15	15	16	18	90th
85th	8	11	12	14	13	14	17	85th
80th	7	10	11	13	12	12	15	80th
75th	6	9	10	12	11	12	14	75th
70th	6	8	9	11	10	11	13	70th
65th	5	7	9	10	9	10	12	65th
60th	5	6	8	9	8	10	11	60th
55th	4	6	7	8	7	9	10	55th
50th	4	5	7	8	6	8	9	50th
45th	3	5	6	7	6	8	9	45th
40th	3	4	6	6	5	7	8	40th
35th	2	4	5	5	4	6	7	35th
30th	2	3	4	5	4	5	6	30th
25th	1	2	4	4	3	5	5	25th
20th	1	2	3	3	2	4	5	20th
15th	0	1	2	3	2	3	4	15th
10th	0	0	2	2	1	2	3	10th
5th	0	0	1	1	0	0	2	5th
0	0	0	0	0	0	0	0	0

Table 2.48

SPEED THROW

Percentile Scores Based on Age / Test Scores in Seconds and Tenths

Percentile	10-11	12	13	14	15	16	17-18	Percentile
				AGE				
100th	13.1	11.0	10.0	9.0	13.0	10.0	10.0	100th
95th	16.1	15.3	14.9	13.0	13.5	12.5	12.1	95th
90th	17.1	16.1	14.9	14.0	13.8	13.2	12.8	90th
85th	17.6	16.8	15.7	14.6	14.2	13.7	13.2	85th
80th	18.0	17.3	16.2	15.1	14.5	14.1	13.3	80th
75th	18.6	17.6	16.8	15.6	14.9	14.5	13.9	75th
70th	19.1	18.0	16.9	15.9	15.6	14.8	14.2	70th
65th	19.7	18.4	17.3	16.3	15.9	15.1	14.5	65th
60th	20.2	18.9	17.6	16.6	16.0	15.5	14.8	60th
55th	20.8	19.5	17.9	17.1	16.4	15.8	14.9	55th
50th	21.3	19.8	18.4	17.3	16.7	16.4	15.3	50th
45th	21.8	20.4	19.1	17.7	17.1	16.6	15.6	45th
40th	22.6	21.0	19.3	18.1	17.5	17.1	16.2	40th
35th	23.6	21.5	19.8	18.5	17.9	17.4	16.7	35th
30th	24.6	22.2	20.6	19.0	18.3	18.2	17.2	30th
25th	25.7	23.1	21.2	19.5	18.9	18.8	17.6	25th
20th	26.7	23.9	21.9	20.2	19.5	19.4	18.3	20th
15th	28.2	25.4	23.0	21.3	20.2	19.9	18.9	15th
10th	30.1	27.8	24.2	22.5	20.9	20.9	19.9	10th
5th	34.7	29.5	26.4	25.1	22.2	23.0	21.2	5th
0	43.1	36.0	29.3	28.2	24.9	25.5	26.1	0

SPEED THROW (GIRLS)

Percentile Scores Based on Age / Test Scores in Seconds and Tenths

Percentile	10-11	12	13	14	15	16	17-18	Percentile
				AGE				
100th	10.0	12.0	12.0	12.0	12.0	14.0	14.0	100th
95th	20.1	13.8	13.0	13.0	15.6	15.8	15.0	95th
90th	21.4	15.8	16.3	13.9	16.6	16.9	15.0	90th
85th	22.8	17.7	17.8	15.3	17.6	17.6	15.6	85th
80th	24.1	18.8	18.6	16.5	18.1	18.1	16.1	80th
75th	25.2	19.8	19.4	17.6	18.6	18.5	17.6	75th
70th	26.0	20.8	20.0	18.2	19.1	18.9	18.0	70th
65th	27.0	21.6	20.6	18.7	19.6	19.4	18.5	65th
60th	27.4	22.3	21.3	19.3	20.1	20.0	18.9	60th
55th	28.8	23.1	21.9	19.9	20.6	20.7	19.3	55th
50th	29.8	24.1	22.7	20.7	21.1	21.4	19.8	50th
45th	30.9	25.2	23.4	21.1	21.7	22.2	20.3	45th
40th	31.9	26.2	24.3	21.8	22.6	22.9	20.8	40th
35th	33.0	27.5	25.4	22.5	23.3	23.7	21.4	35th
30th	34.1	28.6	26.4	23.5	24.3	24.8	22.3	30th
25th	35.9	29.8	27.5	24.6	25.4	26.1	23.3	25th
20th	38.0	31.3	28.9	25.8	26.9	27.8	24.1	20th
15th	41.0	33.1	30.9	27.4	28.7	30.4	25.0	15th
10th	46.1	36.7	33.0	30.2	31.5	33.0	26.1	10th
5th	55.2	40.8	38.5	33.5	37.4	36.9	28.9	5th
0	105.0	66.0	52.0	50.0	50.0	52.0	40.0	0

Table 2.49

FUNGO HITTING

Percentile Scores Based on Age / Test Scores in Points

Percentile	10-11	12	13	14	15	16	17-18	Percentile
100th	40	40	39	36	40	40	40	100th
95th	35	36	38	35	39	38	39	95th
90th	32	33	34	35	37	36	37	90th
85th	29	31	33	33	34	34	36	85th
80th	27	30	31	31	33	33	35	80th
75th	26	29	30	30	31	33	34	75th
70th	24	28	29	29	30	32	32	70th
65th	22	27	28	28	29	30	31	65th
60th	21	26	27	27	28	29	30	60th
55th	20	25	25	26	26	28	29	55th
50th	19	23	24	24	24	26	28	50th
45th	17	22	23	23	23	25	26	45th
40th	16	20	21	21	21	23	25	40th
35th	14	19	19	19	19	21	23	35th
30th	13	17	18	18	17	19	21	30th
25th	11	15	16	16	16	17	19	25th
20th	10	13	15	15	14	15	17	20th
15th	8	11	14	13	12	13	15	15th
10th	6	10	12	12	11	11	13	10th
5th	3	7	9	11	9	9	11	5th
0	0	0	1	9	1	0	3	0

FUNGO HITTING (GIRLS)

Percentile Scores Based on Age / Test Scores in Points

Percentile	10-11	12	13	14	15	16	17-18	Percentile
100th	30	38	38	38	38	38	38	100th
95th	21	28	30	31	30	30	31	95th
90th	18	24	26	30	27	27	28	90th
85th	15	22	23	26	25	25	26	85th
80th	14	20	22	23	23	24	25	80th
75th	13	18	20	21	22	22	23	75th
70th	12	17	19	20	20	21	22	70th
65th	12	16	18	19	19	19	20	65th
60th	11	15	17	18	18	18	19	60th
55th	9	14	16	17	17	17	18	55th
50th	9	13	14	15	16	16	17	50th
45th	8	12	13	14	15	15	16	45th
40th	7	11	13	13	14	14	15	40th
35th	6	10	12	12	13	13	14	35th
30th	6	9	11	11	12	12	14	30th
25th	5	8	10	10	11	11	13	25th
20th	4	7	8	9	10	10	12	20th
15th	3	5	7	8	8	9	10	15th
10th	2	4	6	6	7	8	8	10th
5th	0	2	4	3	4	5	6	5th
0	0	0	0	0	0	0	0	0

156

Table 2.50

BASE RUNNING

Percentile Scores Based on Age / Test Scores in Seconds and Tenths

Percentile	AGE							Percentile
	10-11	12	13	14	15	16	17-18	
100th	10.1	9.6	9.4	9.7	10.0	10.0	10.0	100th
95th	12.9	12.4	11.7	11.5	11.6	11.3	11.1	95th
90th	13.5	12.5	12.2	11.9	11.9	11.6	11.4	90th
85th	13.9	13.3	12.7	12.2	12.2	11.8	11.6	85th
80th	14.1	13.5	12.9	12.5	12.4	12.0	11.8	80th
75th	14.3	13.7	13.2	12.7	12.5	12.1	11.9	75th
70th	14.5	13.9	13.4	12.9	12.7	12.3	12.0	70th
65th	14.8	14.1	13.6	13.0	12.8	12.4	12.2	65th
60th	14.9	14.3	13.8	13.1	13.0	12.5	12.3	60th
55th	15.1	14.5	13.9	13.3	13.1	12.6	12.4	55th
50th	15.2	14.7	14.1	13.4	13.2	12.8	12.6	50th
45th	15.4	14.8	14.3	13.5	13.3	12.9	12.7	45th
40th	15.6	15.0	14.5	13.7	13.5	13.0	12.8	40th
35th	15.8	15.2	14.7	13.9	13.6	13.2	12.9	35th
30th	16.0	15.4	14.9	14.1	13.7	13.3	13.0	30th
25th	16.2	15.7	15.1	14.2	13.9	13.6	13.2	25th
20th	16.5	15.9	15.4	14.5	14.0	13.8	13.4	20th
15th	17.0	16.2	15.7	14.8	14.3	14.1	13.6	15th
10th	17.4	16.5	15.9	15.2	14.5	14.4	13.9	10th
5th	18.2	17.4	16.7	15.8	15.0	15.3	14.9	5th
0	23.0	20.6	17.2	17.2	15.8	18.0	17.8	0

BASE RUNNING (GIRLS)

Percentile Scores Based on Age / Test Scores in Seconds and Tenths

Percentile	AGE							Percentile
	10-11	12	13	14	15	16	17-18	
100th	11.0	11.0	12.0	12.0	12.0	12.0	12.0	100th
95th	13.1	13.4	12.6	12.7	12.9	13.2	13.6	95th
90th	13.8	13.7	13.1	13.1	13.5	13.7	13.9	90th
85th	14.3	14.0	13.5	13.5	13.7	14.0	14.3	85th
80th	14.7	14.3	13.7	13.7	13.9	14.4	14.6	80th
75th	14.9	14.5	13.9	13.8	14.1	14.6	14.8	75th
70th	15.2	14.7	14.1	14.0	14.3	14.8	14.9	70th
65th	15.4	14.9	14.3	14.2	14.5	14.9	15.1	65th
60th	15.6	15.0	14.5	14.4	14.7	15.1	15.3	60th
55th	15.8	15.2	14.7	14.5	14.9	15.3	15.5	55th
50th	16.0	15.3	14.8	14.8	15.0	15.5	15.7	50th
45th	16.2	15.5	15.0	14.9	15.2	15.6	15.9	45th
40th	16.4	15.7	15.2	15.1	15.4	15.8	16.1	40th
35th	16.7	15.8	15.4	15.3	15.5	15.9	16.3	35th
30th	17.0	16.0	15.6	15.5	15.8	16.0	16.5	30th
25th	17.3	16.2	16.0	15.7	16.1	16.2	16.9	25th
20th	17.7	16.5	16.3	16.0	16.3	16.3	17.1	20th
15th	18.2	16.9	16.6	16.4	16.7	16.4	17.6	15th
10th	18.8	17.4	17.2	16.9	17.3	17.8	18.2	10th
5th	19.9	18.2	18.0	17.8	18.1	18.4	19.2	5th
0	27.0	20.0	22.0	23.0	28.0	31.0	32.0	0

Table 2.51

FIELDING GROUND BALLS

Percentile Scores Based on Age / Test Scores in Points

Percentile	AGE							Percentile
	10-11	12	13	14	15	16	17-18	
100th	20	20	20	20	20	20	20	100th
95th	19	20	20	20	20	20	20	95th
90th	18	19	19	19	19	20	20	90th
85th	18	19	19	19	19	20	20	85th
80th	17	18	18	18	18	19	19	80th
75th	17	18	18	18	18	19	19	75th
70th	16	17	17	17	18	19	19	70th
65th	16	17	17	17	17	18	18	65th
60th	15	16	16	16	16	18	18	60th
55th	15	16	16	16	16	17	17	55th
50th	14	15	15	15	15	17	17	50th
45th	13	15	14	14	15	16	17	45th
40th	13	14	14	14	14	16	16	40th
35th	12	14	13	13	13	15	16	35th
30th	11	13	13	12	12	14	15	30th
25th	10	12	12	10	11	13	14	25th
20th	9	11	11	10	10	10	12	20th
15th	8	9	10	9	9	9	10	15th
10th	6	8	8	8	8	9	9	10th
5th	4	6	6	6	7	8	9	5th
0	0	0	1	1	1	5	6	0

FIELDING GROUND BALLS (GIRLS)

Percentile Scores Based on Age / Test Scores in Points

Percentile	AGE							Percentile
	10-11	12	13	14	15	16	17-18	
100th	20	20	20	20	20	20	20	100th
95th	18	20	20	20	20	20	20	95th
90th	17	19	19	19	20	20	20	90th
85th	16	19	19	19	19	19	19	85th
80th	15	18	19	19	19	19	19	80th
75th	15	18	18	18	18	19	19	75th
70th	14	17	18	17	18	18	18	70th
65th	13	16	17	17	18	18	18	65th
60th	13	15	17	17	17	18	18	60th
55th	12	15	16	17	17	17	17	55th
50th	11	14	16	16	16	17	17	50th
45th	10	13	15	15	16	17	17	45th
40th	10	12	15	15	15	16	16	40th
35th	9	10	14	14	15	16	16	35th
30th	8	10	13	13	14	15	15	30th
25th	8	9	12	12	13	14	14	25th
20th	7	9	11	10	12	13	14	20th
15th	6	8	10	10	11	12	13	15th
10th	5	7	9	9	10	10	11	10th
5th	3	5	8	8	9	8	9	5th
0	0	0	0	0	0	0	0	0

Table 2.52

CATCHING FLY BALLS
Percentile Scores Based on Age / Test Scores in Points

Percentile	10-11	12	13	14	15	16	17-18	Percentile
100th	20	20	20	20	20	20	20	100th
95th	20	20	20	20	20	20	20	95th
90th	20	20	20	20	20	20	20	90th
85th	19	19	19	19	20	20	20	85th
80th	19	19	19	19	19	19	19	80th
75th	19	19	19	19	19	19	19	75th
70th	18	19	18	19	19	19	19	70th
65th	18	18	18	18	18	19	19	65th
60th	17	18	17	18	18	18	18	60th
55th	17	17	17	18	17	18	18	55th
50th	16	17	16	16	17	17	18	50th
45th	15	16	16	16	16	16	17	45th
40th	14	15	15	15	15	15	16	40th
35th	12	14	14	13	14	13	15	35th
30th	10	12	13	12	12	10	14	30th
25th	9	10	11	10	11	10	11	25th
20th	8	10	10	10	10	10	10	20th
15th	7	8	9	9	9	9	10	15th
10th	6	7	8	8	8	9	9	10th
5th	3	5	6	7	7	8	9	5th
0	0	0	0	0	0	0	0	0

CATCHING FLY BALLS (GIRLS)
Percentile Scores Based on Age / Test Scores in Points

Percentile	10-11	12	13	14	15	16	17-18	Percentile
100th	15	17	19	19	20	20	20	100th
95th	13	15	17	17	19	19	19	95th
90th	10	13	15	16	18	19	19	90th
85th	9	11	13	15	18	18	18	85th
80th	9	10	12	14	17	17	17	80th
75th	8	9	11	13	16	16	16	75th
70th	7	8	10	12	15	15	16	70th
65th	7	7	9	11	14	14	15	65th
60th	6	7	8	10	13	13	15	60th
55th	6	6	7	9	12	13	14	55th
50th	5	6	6	9	11	12	13	50th
45th	4	5	5	8	10	11	12	45th
40th	4	5	5	8	9	10	11	40th
35th	3	4	4	7	8	9	10	35th
30th	3	3	3	6	7	8	9	30th
25th	2	3	3	5	6	7	8	25th
20th	2	2	2	4	5	6	7	20th
15th	1	2	2	3	4	5	6	15th
10th	1	1	1	2	3	4	5	10th
5th	0	0	0	1	2	3	4	5th
0	0	0	0	0	0	0	0	0

SWIMMING SKILL TESTS

Wilson Achievement Test for Intermediate Swimming*

Floor Plan and Space Requirements

A 75-foot pool is required and the norms reported pertain to a pool of this size.

Test Description

ITEM NUMBER I—TIME: 25-YARD FLUTTER KICK
WITH KICKBOARD

Purpose

To measure speed of flutter kick.

Facilities and Equipment

Stop watch, 25-yard distance in pool or lake—no current.

Procedures

The swimmer's partner holds her ankles with the pointed toes brushing the end of the pool. The swimmer is fully extended in a prone position holding a flutter board at arms' length. The partner is on the deck. The feet are released as the signal is given to begin kicking. The Hewitt test permits the swimmer to push-off and to hold a water polo ball.

Instructions

"Hold the flutter board at arms' length and be prepared to go the length of the pool using your flutter kick. Your partner will hold your ankles just under the surface of the water until the signal to 'Go!' Kick until your flutter board hits the opposite end of the pool and get there as quickly as possible."

Scoring

The score is the number of seconds required to cover the 25 yards. No push-off is permitted. The partner who was holding the ankles walks down the side of the pool to be at the end when the swimmer arrives. She listens for the call of the seconds by the instructor to learn the correct second when her partner's flutter board touched the end. She reports the time to the instructor.

---

*Wilson, Marcia Ruth, "A Relationship Between General Motor Ability and Objective Measures of Achievement in Swimming at the Intermediate Level for College Women," unpublished Master's Thesis, The Women's College of the University of North Carolina, Greensboro, 1962. Used by permission of the author.

Testing Personnel

A partner for each swimmer. A central timer who calls out the seconds as the swimmers approach the end of the pool and who also records the scores.

ITEM NUMBER II—TIME: 25-YARD SCULLING

Purpose

To measure ability to progress through the water using only the arms in a sculling pattern.

Facilities and Equipment

Twenty five-yard pool, stop watch.

Procedures

The swimmer assumes a back position with the toes barely touching the end of the pool. A partner holds the ankles just under the surface of the water. At the end of the 25-yard distance, the partner, who has walked to the other end of the pool, places the back of her hand against the end of the pool with the palm open to receive the swimmer's head. Time is taken at the instant of contact.

Instructions

"Get on your back ready to scull. Your partner will hold your ankles until you are ready to begin. On the signal, 'Ready, Go!' scull as fast as possible to the other end of the pool. Do not use any kicking actions. You will be timed from the start until your head contacts your partner's hand at the other end of the pool."

Scoring

The score is the number of seconds required to scull 25 yards. The partner listens to the seconds called out by the instructor and reports the one just called as the swimmer's head contacts her hand. The partner, who walks down the side of the pool, watches for any kicking motions and disqualifies the trial if they occur.

Testing Personnel

A central timer and a partner who checks for fouls, scores, and assists at the beginning and the end of the test.

ITEM NUMBER III—NUMBER OF STROKES: 25-YARD SIDE STROKE

Purpose

To measure the power of the side stroke and the efficiency of the glide.

Facilities and Equipment

Twenty five-yard pool.

Procedures

The partner starts the swimmer at the end of the pool holding her ankles 6 to 8 inches under the water in the side position. When the swimmer is ready, the partner releases her ankles and walks along the side of the pool counting each power phase of the stroke.

Note: The Hewitt tests of power for the elementary back stroke, side stroke and breast stroke permit a push-off which is counted as 1 stroke.

Instructions

"Assume a position for the side stroke with your glide arms fully extended. Your partner will hold your ankles until you indicate to her that you are ready to swim. Perform the side stroke for the length of the pool using as few strokes as possible. Each power phase of the stroke will count as one stroke."

Scoring

Score 1 stroke for every power phase of the side stroke performed by the swimmer. The regulation scissor kick is required. Report the score to the instructor.

Testing Personnel

A partner for each swimmer and a central recorder for the entire class.

ITEM NUMBER IV—DISTANCE IN FEET:
PLUNGE DIVE AND GLIDE

Purpose

To measure ability to perform a plunge dive and to achieve distance on the glide.

Facilities and Equipment

A swimming pool marked at 5-foot intervals along one side of the deck.

Procedures

The swimmer performs a plunge dive and glides as far as possible. The dive should occur in the first lane in close proximity to the marked distances.

Instructions

"Please dive into the first lane and glide as far as you can. I will measure the distance when you surface to the point where your fingers break the water. No arm pull or kick is permitted."

Scoring

The score is the distance in feet measured to the point where the fingers first surface.

Testing Personnel

One person to spot the distance and record the score.

ITEM NUMBER V—UNDERWATER SWIM

Purpose

To measure breath control and ability to stay under water and to make progress under water.

Facilities and Equipment

Seven bricks with numbers painted on 6 of them, a width of pool space approximately of 2 lanes and about 40 feet in length, water of from 4 to 7 feet in depth.

Procedures

The swimmer stands in 4-foot water with her toes behind the brick. She takes a breath and swims under water, turning as many bricks as possible in the numbered order. Each brick is turned 1/4 turn.

Instructions

"Stand behind the starting brick and, when you are ready, push off into a front surface dive. Swim under water to each brick following the numbers painted on the bricks and turn each brick 1/4 turn. See how many bricks you can turn before you have to surface."

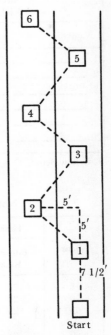

Figure 2.59. Specifications for the Underwater Swim Test.

Scoring

The instructor or partner can score from the deck of the pool by observing the number of bricks turned. The score is the number of bricks turned, while swimming under water on one breath of air. If the majority of the students can score 6, have them start on the return trip to the starting brick and continue adding the number of bricks turned.

Testing Personnel

A scorer and recorder. Occasionally, someone has to re-set the bricks on their original spots. This is not necessary after each trial.

Score Card

WILSON INTERMEDIATE SWIMMING TESTS

Names	Time 25-yd. Flutter Kick		Time 25-yd. Scull		Strokes 25-yd. Side Stroke		Feet Dive and Glide		Turns Underwater Swim	
	R	T	R	T	R	T	R	T	R	T
1.										
2.										
3.										
.										
.										
20.										

R = Raw Score, T = T-Score

Table 2.53

Norms for Wilson Intermediate Swimming Tests*

T-Score	Time Flutter Kick	Time Sculling	Strokes Side Stroke	Feet Plunge Dive	Turns Underwater Swim	T-Score
75	22	35		33	6	75
70	24	37	7	32		70
65	25	41		31		65
60	28	45	6	29		60
55	29	50	9	26	5	55
50	34	54	10	25	4	50
45	38	59	12	23	3	45
40	42	65	15	20	2	40
35	56	74	17	16	1	35
30	76	83	21	15		30
25	100	89	33			25

*Based on the performance of 70 college women.

TENNIS SKILL TEST

Backboard Test of Tennis Ability*
Revised Directions

Equipment

1. Backboard or wall, approximately ten feet in height and allowing about fifteen feet in width per person taking the test at one time. Two players taking the test at once has been found to be a very satisfactory arrangement. This allows for adequate supervision by the administrator.

TABLE 2.54
T Scale For New Method Scoring

T Scale	Test Score	T Scale	Test Score	T Scale	Test Score	T Scale	Test Score
100	67	75	50	50	33	25	16
99	66	74	49	49	32	24	15
98		73		48		23	
97	65	72	48	47	31	22	14
96	64	71	47	46	30	21	13
95		70		45		20	
94	63	69	46	44	29	19	12
93	62	68	45	43	28	18	11
92		67	44	42	27	17	10
91	61	66		41		16	
90	60	65	43	40	26	15	9
89	59	64	42	39	25	14	8
88		63		38		13	
87	58	62	41	37	24	12	7
86	57	61	40	36	23	11	6
85		60		35		10	
84	56	59	38	34	22	9	5
83	55	58	39	33	21	8	4
82		57		32		7	
81	54	56	37	31	20	6	3
80	53	55	36	30	19	5	2
79		54		29		4	
78	52	53	35	28	18	3	1
77	51	52	24	27	17	2	
76		51		26		1	

*Dyer, Joanna Thayer, "Revision of Backboard Test of Tennis Ability," *Research Quarterly,* Volume 9, No. 1, March, 1938, page 25. Used by permission of the AAHPER.

2. On this wall a plainly visible line three inches in width, to represent the net, should be drawn so that the top is three feet from the ground.

3. A restraining line, five feet from the base of the wall, should be drawn on the floor.*

4. Stop watch with second hand.

5. Two balls and a racquet per player. It is desirable that the balls be in good condition, although it is not essential that they be exactly new. The racquet should be without flaws.

6. Box for extra balls, about 12 inches long, 9 inches wide and 3 inches deep, placed on the floor where the restraining line joins the side at the left for right-handed players and right for left-handed players.

7. One pencil per group of four players.

8. Score card per player.

Organization

Divide the group to be tested into units of four players each, and number them from one to four. Provide each player with a score card on which she writes her name. Then read the following description of the test to the group.

"The Backboard Test consists in rallying a tennis ball against the wall. The object of the test is to cause the ball to strike the wall on or above the net line as many times as you can in 30 seconds. (Pause) When I say 'Go!' start the test immediately. Drop the ball and let it hit the floor once, then put it in play against the wall. Continue to play it to the wall until I say, 'Stop!' at the end of 30 seconds. There is no limit to the number of times the ball may bounce before you hit it. You may volley the ball. The ball need not touch the floor before you play it except at the start and when a new ball is being put in play. You may use any stroke or combination of strokes. You must play all balls from behind this restraining line (indicate the line clearly). You may cross the line to retrieve balls, but any hits made while in such a position do not count. You may use any number of balls. If for any reason you lose control of the ball in play, do not try to retrieve it. Take another ball from this box (indicate clearly) and put it in play as you did at the start. Each ball striking the wall on or above the net line before the word 'Stop' counts as a hit and scores

---

*Hewitt *(69)* revised the Dyer test by extending the restraining line to twenty feet and initiating each rally with a serve. Validities ranged from .68 to .73 for beginners, and .84 to .89 with advanced students. Hewitt believes his revision to be superior with beginning students.

one point. You will each be given three trials today. The final score on the test is the sum of the scores on the three trials."

Demonstrate the following points:

1. Two balls in hand.

2. Start test by dropping ball, letting it hit floor at least once, then play it.

3. Rally a few times, showing volley.

4. Cross restraining line to retrieve a ball, a low hit to keep it in play and retreat for next shot.

5. Make a wild shot to show how taking another ball saves time. Put this new ball in play as at the start.

Read the following paragraph, making certain that each person understands the test procedure and her duties.

"In each group:

"No. 1 takes the test. At the signal, 'Ready?' she stands anywhere behind the restraining line with her racquet and *two balls* prepared to start the test at the word 'Go!'

"No. 2 counts the number of balls which strike the wall on or above the net line *before* the word 'Stop!' and enters them on the score card opposite the appropriate trial number. If any infringements are reported by No. 3 these are deducted before the score for the trial is recorded. A ball striking coincident with the word 'Stop!' does not count.

"No. 3 watches the player in relation to the restraining line. She reports to the scorer at the end of the trial the number of hits, if any, made while the player was standing closer to the wall than the restraining line.

"No. 4 collects the balls of her group before the start of a trial and puts them in the box. During the trial she collects and returns to the box any balls going out of play.

"Each person takes the test in rotation. After No. 1 has had her first trials she assumes the duties of No. 2 while the latter takes the test; No. 3 and No. 4 remain the same. While No. 3 takes the test, No. 4 scores the hits, No. 1 and No. 2 assume the duties of No. 3 and No. 4 respectively. When No. 4 takes the test, No. 3 scores hits, and No. 1 and No. 2 remain the same. After each person in the entire group being tested has had one trial, the test is repeated in the same order until everyone has had three trials in all."

Answer questions. This organization will consume about ten minutes. Great care should be exercised in these preliminaries to make certain that the test procedure is clearly understood. The testing will then take place smoothly and accurately.

The examiner then assumes a position to the rear of the players with the stop watch, and begins testing the No. 1's who are to take the test at one time, usually one or two. Numbers 2, 3, and 4 of these groups will follow, and then the No. 1 of the next two groups, and so on until all have had one trial, after which the test is repeated twice in the same order. In case the group does not divide exactly into groups of four, adjust groups to suit.

VOLLEYBALL SKILL TESTS*
VOLLEYING

Purpose

To measure ability and speed with which a player can volley a volleyball against a wall.

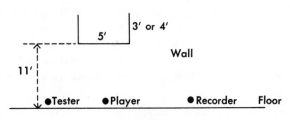

Figure 2.60.

Equipment

A solid smooth wall with a one-inch wide line marked on it which is five feet long and is 11 feet above and parallel to the floor and vertical lines extending upward from each end of the line that are three or four feet long, volleyball, stop watch, scoring sheet.

Description

The player with volleyball in hand stands facing the wall. On signal "go" the ball is tossed against the wall into the area bounded by the

*AAHPER, *Volleyball Skills Test Manual,* Washington, D.C. American Association for Health, Physical Education, and Recreation, (1201 16th St. N.W., Washington, D.C.). Used by permission of the AAHPER.

lines. On the rebound the ball is then volleyed into the marked area and is continued to be volleyed consecutively for one minute.

Rules

1. The ball is held in the hands prior to the toss at start of the test.
2. The tossed ball and each volley must strike the wall above the five-foot line and between the two vertical lines.
3. On a miss or a catch the test continues by the player again tossing the ball against the wall and volleying on the rebound.
4. The player continues to toss and/or volley until the expiration of one minute.

Scoring

Score is the total number of legal volleys executed within one minute. Tosses do not count in the score. Scores above 50 are not recorded.

SERVING

Purpose

To measure the player's skill in serving as in an acutal game.

Equipment

Volleyballs, volleyball net and standards, court marked as indicated in diagram.

Description

Server X stands opposite the marked court in the proper serving position. He may use any legal serve in hitting the ball over the net

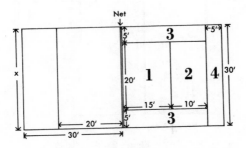

Figure 2.61.

into the opposite court. For children below the age of 12, the serving line should be located 20 feet from the net.

Rules

1. The server is given ten trials.
2. When the ball hits the net and does or does not go over, it counts as a trial but no points are given.

Scoring

The score is the total number of points made, determined by where the ball lands in the opposite court. For all balls that strike on a line, the higher score of the areas concerned is awarded with 40 the maximum.

PASSING

Purpose

To measure the player's skill in passing a volleyball from the rear of the court toward the net.

Equipment

Volleyballs, volleyball net and standards, four-foot by six-foot mats or marked areas on floor, 30-foot rope and two standards eight feet high.

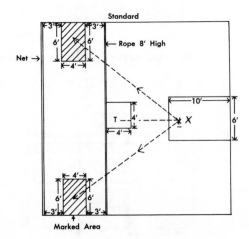

Figure 2.62.

Description

Passer X—person being tested—stands in center back position of court, receives a high throw (similar to two-hand basketball shot) from thrower T, and executes a pass so that it goes over the rope and onto the mat or marked area.

Rules

1. Passer is given 20 trials performed alternately to the right and to the left.
2. The trial counts but no points are recorded if ball touches rope or net, or does not fall on target area.

Scoring

One point is scored for each pass going over the rope and landing on or hitting any part of the target area (including lines) with 20 the maximum.

SET-UP

Purpose

To measure the player's ability to set-up the volleyball toward the net.

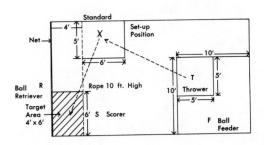

Figure 2.63.

Equipment

Volleyballs, volleyball net and standards, four-foot by six-foot mats or marked areas on floor, 30-foot rope and two standards—ten feet high for boys and nine feet high for girls.

Description

Set-up man X stands in mid-court position within the six-foot by five-foot area as shown. He receives a high throw (similar to two-hand basketball shot) from thrower T, and executes a set-up so that it goes over the rope and onto the target area. Two subjects may be tested simultaneously, one setting up the ball to the right and the other to the left.

Rules

1. Throws from T that do not fall into the six-foot by five-foot area are to be repeated.
2. Set-up man has ten trials to the right and ten to the left.
3. The trial counts but no points are recorded if the ball touches rope or net, or does not fall on the target area.

Scoring

One point is scored for each set-up that goes over the rope and lands on or hits any part of the target area (including lines) with 20 the maximum.

Table 2.55

VOLLEYING TEST (BOYS)
Percentile Scores Based on Age / Test Scores in Points

Percentile	10-11	12	13	14	15	16	17-18	Percentile
100	40	42	44	50	50	50	50	100
95	24	31	35	39	42	44	45	95
90	19	28	30*	36	40	41	42	90
85	17	24	28	33	36	38	42	85
80	15	22	26	31	34	36	41	80
75	13	19	24	29	32	34	40	75
70	12	18	22	27	30	33	39	70
65	11	17	21	26	29	32	37	65
60	9	16	19	24	28	30	36	60
55	8	15	18	23	27	28	34	55
50	7	13	17	21	25	26	32	50
45	6	12	15	19	24	25	29	45
40	5	11	14	18	22	23	27	40
35	4	9	12	17	20	21	24	35
30	3	8	11	15	18	19	23	30
25	3	7	9	13	17	18	20	25
20	2	6	8	11	15	16	19	20
15	1	4	7	9	13	15	17	15
10	0	3	5	7	10	12	14	10
5	0	2	3	5	6	11	11	5
0	0	0	0	0	0	0	0	0

VOLLEYING TEST (GIRLS)
Percentile Scores Based on Age / Test Scores in Points

Percentile	10-11	12	13	14	15	16	17-18	Percentile
100	47	49	49	50	50	50	50	100
95	21	29	31	32	37	40	40	95
90	13	24	25	26	31	36	38	90
85	10	19	20	21	24	28	31	85
80	8	16	17	19	21	25	27	80
75	6	13	15	17	18	22	23	75
70	5	11	13	14	16	20	20	70
65	4	10	11	13	15	18	18	65
60	3	8	10	12	13	16	16	60
55	3	7	9	11	12	14	14	55
50	2	6	8	10	11	12	12	50
45	2	5	7	9	10	11	11	45
40	1	4	6	8	9	9	9	40
35	1	3	5	7	8	8	8	35
30	1	2	4	6	7	7	7	30
25	0	2	3	5	6	6	6	25
20	0	1	1	4	5	5	5	20
15	0	1	1	3	4	4	4	15
10	0	0	0	1	2	3	3	10
5	0	0	0	0	1	2	2	5
0	0	0	0	0	0	0	0	0

Table 2.56

SERVING TEST (BOYS)

Percentile Scores Based on Age / Test Scores in Points

Percentile	10-11	12	13	14	15	16	17-18	Percentile
100	39	40	40	40	40	40	40	100
95	29	31	32	34	36	37	37	95
90	27	28	29	31	33	33	33	90
85	25	26	27	29	32	32	32	85
80	23	24	26	27	30	30	31	80
75	22	23	24	25	28	29	30	75
70	21	21	23	24	28	29	30	70
65	20	20	22	23	27	28	29	65
60	18	19	21	22	25	27	27	60
55	17	18	20	21	24	25	26	55
50	16	16	19	20	22	23	24	50
45	15	15	18	19	21	22	22	45
40	14	14	17	18	20	21	21	40
35	13	13	16	17	19	19	20	35
30	12	12	15	16	18	19	19	30
25	11	11	13	15	16	17	17	25
20	9	10	12	14	15	15	16	20
15	8	9	10	12	12	13	14	15
10	7	8	8	10	11	12	12	10
5	4	5	5	8	9	10	11	5
0	0	3	3	5	6	6	7	0

SERVING TEST (GIRLS)

Percentile Scores Based on Age / Test Scores in Points

Percentile	10-11	12	13	14	15	16	17-18	Percentile
100	36	38	40	40	40	40	40	100
95	24	26	26	28	30	31	32	95
90	20	22	23	26	26	26	26	90
85	18	20	20	23	23	24	24	85
80	16	18	18	21	21	22	23	80
75	15	16	17	20	20	21	21	75
70	14	15	15	18	19	20	20	70
65	13	14	14	17	17	19	19	65
60	12	13	13	15	16	18	18	60
55	11	12	12	14	15	17	17	55
50	10	11	11	13	14	16	16	50
45	9	10	10	11	13	15	15	45
40	8	9	9	10	12	14	14	40
35	7	8	8	9	11	13	14	35
30	6	6	7	8	10	13	13	30
25	5	5	5	7	9	11	11	25
20	4	4	4	6	8	10	10	20
15	2	3	3	5	6	8	9	15
10	1	1	1	3	4	7	7	10
5	0	0	0	1	2	4	4	5
0	0	0	0	0	0	0	0	0

Table 2.57

PASSING TEST (BOYS)
Percentile Scores Based on Age / Test Scores in Points

Percentile	10-11	12	13	14	15	16	17-18	Percentile
100	19	19	19	20	20	20	20	100
95	12	14	16	17	17	17	17	95
90	10	13	14	16	16	16	16	90
85	9	12	13	15	15	15	15	85
80	8	11	12	14	14	14	14	80
75	7	10	12	13	13	13	13	75
70	6	9	11	12	12	12	13	70
65	5	8	10	12	12	12	13	65
60	4	8	9	11	11	12	12	60
55	4	7	9	10	10	12	12	55
50	3	6	8	10	10	11	11	50
45	3	5	7	9	9	10	10	45
40	2	4	7	8	8	9	9	40
35	2	4	6	8	8	9	9	35
30	1	3	5	7	7	8	8	30
25	1	2	4	6	6	7	8	25
20	0	2	4	5	5	6	7	20
15	0	1	3	4	4	5	6	15
10	0	0	2	3	3	4	4	10
5	0	0	1	2	2	2	2	5
0	0	0	0	0	0	2	0	0

PASSING TEST (GIRLS)
Percentile Scores Based on Age / Test Scores in Points

Percentile	10-11	12	13	14	15	16	17-18	Percentile
100	19	19	20	20	20	20	20	100
95	10	12	12	13	13	14	15	95
90	8	10	10	11	11	12	13	90
85	7	8	9	10	10	11	12	85
80	6	7	8	9	9	10	11	80
75	5	6	7	8	8	8	9	75
70	4	6	6	7	7	8	9	70
65	3	5	5	6	6	8	8	65
60	3	4	4	6	6	7	8	60
55	2	4	4	5	5	6	7	55
50	2	3	4	5	5	6	6	50
45	1	3	3	4	4	5	6	45
40	1	2	3	4	4	4	5	40
35	0	2	2	3	3	4	4	35
30	0	1	2	3	3	3	4	30
25	0	1	1	2	2	3	3	25
20	0	0	1	1	2	2	3	20
15	0	0	0	1	1	2	2	15
10	0	0	0	0	1	1	1	10
5	0	0	0	0	0	0	0	5
0	0	0	0	0	0	0	0	0

Table 2.58

SET-UP TEST (BOYS)
Percentile Scores Based on Age / Test Scores in Points

Percentile	10-11	12	13	14	15	16	17-18	Percentile
100	16	18	20	20	20	20	20	100
95	10	14	16	16	16	17	17	95
90	9	12	14	15	15	15	15	90
85	8	11	13	13	13	14	15	85
80	7	10	12	12	12	13	14	80
75	6	9	11	11	11	12	13	75
70	6	8	10	10	10	10	11	70
65	5	8	9	9	9	9	11	65
60	5	7	8	8	8	9	10	60
55	4	7	7	8	8	8	10	55
50	4	6	7	7	7	7	9	50
45	3	6	6	6	6	6	9	45
40	3	5	6	6	6	6	8	40
35	3	5	5	5	5	5	7	35
30	2	4	4	5	5	5	7	30
25	2	4	4	4	4	4	6	25
20	2	3	3	4	4	4	6	20
15	1	3	3	3	3	3	5	15
10	0	1	1	2	2	2	2	10
5	0	1	1	1	1	1	2	5
0	0	0	0	0	0	0	1	0

SET-UP TEST (GIRLS)
Percentile Scores Based on Age / Test Scores in Points

Percentile	10-11	12	13	14	15	16	17-18	Percentile
100	19	20	20	20	20	20	20	100
95	11	13	14	14	14	15	15	95
90	9	11	11	12	12	12	14	90
85	7	9	10	10	11	11	12	85
80	6	8	9	10	10	10	11	80
75	5	7	8	9	9	9	10	75
70	5	6	7	8	8	8	8	70
65	4	6	7	7	7	7	7	65
60	4	5	6	6	6	7	7	60
55	3	5	5	6	6	6	6	55
50	3	4	5	5	5	6	6	50
45	2	4	4	4	4	5	5	45
40	2	3	4	4	4	5	5	40
35	2	3	3	3	3	4	4	35
30	1	2	3	3	3	3	4	30
25	1	2	2	2	2	3	3	25
20	1	2	2	2	1	2	3	20
15	0	1	1	1	1	2	2	15
10	0	0	1	1	1	1	1	10
5	0	0	0	0	0	1	1	5
0	0	0	0	0	0	0	0	0

Game Performance Testing

Most game performance must be tested through subjective evaluation but this can be made more objective with rating scales. It would be unfair to grade a single player solely on the tournament standing of his team, since team performance is the result of the efforts and abilities of all the players, not of any one player.

One instrument has been devised which proves valid and is based on the evaluation by team members of each other team member. This instrument is included here. For further help in team-play evaluation see sections on rating scales and grading.

No. _____ Item _____   Person being rated_____
                                                                    (last name first)

                                                 Rater_____

**THE BELMONT MEASURES
OF ATHLETIC PERFORMANCE**

Basketball

Basketball Scale for Women

Copyrighted 1964

Logan Wright
George Peabody College for Teachers
and
Patsy K. Wright
Belmont College

1. ☐☐ Is a poor sport.
Does not know the rules of the game.

2. ☐☐ Is alert at all times.
Is not rough or quick-tempered.

3. ☐ Is willing to let some-one take her place if she is not doing well.
☐ Has desire to win.

4. ☐ Knows opponents' weak-nesses.
☐ Is tall.

5. ☐☐ Has sense of humor.
Loves the game.

6. ☐☐ Avoids long passes.
Has a lot of energy.

7. ☐☐ Has big hands.
Is clumsy.

8. ☐ Seldom tires before the game is over.
☐ Has a lot of playing experience.

9. ☐☐.Frequently takes her eyes off the ball.
☐ Reacts slowly.

10. ☐☐ Shoots a lot.
The person guarded often scores.

    Print the name of the person you are rating, last name first, in the space provided for this purpose on each answer sheet. You have a separate answer sheet for each person you are rating. Write a separate name at the top of each answer sheet. Do this now.

    Print your own name, last name first, in the space entitled "rater" on each answer sheet.

    Below are two sample questions. Read the two statements in each sample and decide which one is most characteristic of the first person you are going to rate. Place an X on your answer sheet in the space in front of the item which best describes that person. It is possible that both items are very descriptive of that person or that neither item is very descriptive of her. Your job is to decide, or guess if necessary, which item is most like the person. You must mark one, but only one, of each pair of items. Now do the samples.

    I. ☐ Is a poor sport.
    ☐ Does not know the rules of the game.

    II. ☐ Is alert at all times.
    ☐ Is not rough or quick-tempered.

    Are there questions about the samples? You should have placed one X in the first pair of boxes and another X in the second pair of boxes.

    Throughout the test, the two items in each pair are equally favor-able. It is therefore of no advantage to try to figure out which item is the "best" answer. Rating in this manner could easily harm the person be-ing rated more than it would help her. Instead, you should work quickly and mark items on the basis of which is more characteristic of the person in question.

    At the left there are more pairs of questions. Read each statement carefully and place an X in front of the item in each pair which best des-cribes the person you are rating. Make sure your answers are heavy and black. Erase completely any answer you wish to change.

    After you complete your rating of the first person on your list, proceed on to the next, rating her in the same manner. Continue without waiting for further instructions until all persons on your list have been rated. Be sure to mark one, but only one, of the items in each pair. When you finish a sheet, go immediately to the next. If you have questions, raise your hand.

PSYCHOMETRIC **A**FFILIATES
1743 Monterey
Chicago, Illinois 60643

Basketball Scale for Women

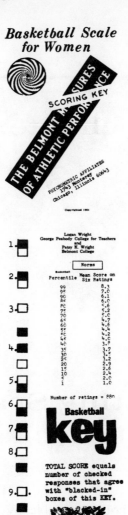

SCORING KEY

THE BELMONT MEASURES OF ATHLETIC PERFORMANCE

PSYCHOMETRIC AFFILIATES
1743 Monterey
Chicago, Illinois 60643

Copyrighted 1964

Logan Wright
George Peabody College for Teachers
and
Patsy K. Wright
Belmont College

Norms

Basketball Percentile	Mean Score on Six Ratings
99	8.3
95	7.0
90	6.1
85	6.0
80	5.6
75	5.2
70	5.0
65	4.7
60	4.4
55	4.2
50	4.0
45	3.8
35	3.7
30	3.5
25	3.2
20	2.9
15	2.6
10	2.4
5	2.0
1	1.0

Number of ratings = 880

Basketball key

TOTAL SCORE equals number of checked responses that agree with "blacked-in" boxes of this KEY.

PSYCHOMETRIC AFFILIATES

chapter

3

Rating Scales
and Check Lists

Some qualities are not measurable by strictly objective means. These include most of the concomitants such as social behavior, some facets of performance such as the quality of execution of a tennis stroke as opposed to accuracy, game play, and some performances such as gymnastics and diving. These are qualities which we must evaluate through subjective ratings. Any time we look at a performance and give a grade, we are making a subjective evaluation; and whether or not we are aware of it, we are using a rating scale. We have in mind certain degrees of excellence in the performance, and these mental pictures are composed of descriptive ideas of the component parts of the performance.

Rating scales are means of objectifying subjective evaluations, of assigning quantitative values to qualitative judgments; whereas check lists are not designed to provide a quantitative evaluation, although they may be used as such, and certainly they become an integral part in the construction of rating scales. A rating scale may be used to evaluate the elements involved in a sport; for example, in golf, one might wish to evaluate use of woods and irons, pitch, chip, putt, and playing different lies, whereas in a checklist each of these elements is broken down into its components.

Example: grip, stance, backswing, pivot, forward swing, contact, and follow through.

One could, of course, assign a value to each component in which case the check list becomes a rating scale; but normally a check list is scored "yes" or "no" on each descriptive phase of a component, or on each component.

How detailed one makes a check list is a matter of preference determined by need. Check lists are very valuable as aids in the learning process to help the student become aware, not only of the factors involved in the skill, but his present status and what he needs to work on.

We have already seen check lists and rating scales used to evaluate social efficiency and posture. There are many rating scales and check lists also devised for use in evaluating performance. One example of each will be presented here, and the student is referred to the bibliography.

EXAMPLE 6

GOLF SWING CHECK LIST DESCRIPTIONS

GRIP
Left-palm, firm; V to right shoulder
Right-finger, V to right shoulder

STANCE
Club head soled, knees relaxed, feet square, left foot turned slightly out, ball off left heel, head down, weight and width of stance appropriate to club

WRISTS
Slightly cocked at address, cocked at extension of back swing but held firmly, uncocked at low point of swing; work together

RIGHT ARM AND SHOULDER
Elbow in, shoulder slightly lower, elbow points to ground at top of backswing

LEFT ARM
Straight until end of follow through
Slight pronation
Pull on forward swing

BACKSWING
  Low until pivot brings it up
  Head over ball
  Pivot in body, no weight shift
  Full pivot

FORWARD SWING
  Starts with left arm pull
  Weight shifts to left
  Head remains over ball
  Wrists remain cocked until bottom of swing
  Stance as at address on contact

POWER AND TIMING
  Clubhead speed at contact
  Wrists come to extension at contact
  Left hand firm, right hand guides

FOLLOW THROUGH
  Low until pivot brings up in line of intended flight
  Head remains in position

GOLF SWING CHECK LIST

Class _____

Time _____

STUDENT	GRIP	STANCE	WRISTS	RT. ARM & SHOULDER	LEFT ARM	BACKSWING	FORWARD SWING	POWER & TIMING	FOLLOW THROUGH
1. _____									
2. _____									
3. _____									
4. _____									
5. _____									

These essentials are the things which are looked for when checking the elements. It is easy to see how the check list might be used in final evaluation, for a student achieving all of the elements should have a better swing than one with some blanks on the check list; however, it should be pointed out that in spite of detailed analysis, the final result involves a quality which is more than the sum of its parts. Some factors are more important than others, and two students with the same number of checks, although on different elements, might well have different degrees of success. For example, Jim might not achieve a full pivot, but make excellent contact with the ball, while Bob, with a full pivot, fails to achieve good timing at contact and consistently smothers the ball. Jim in this case has a more successful swing than does Bob. In the final analysis, ratings must be made on the total element.

EXAMPLE 7A

GOLF RATING SCALE

Woods and Irons

7   *Excellent*—Full swing, coordination and timing consistently produces full speed at contact, flight of ball straight, trajectory appropriate to club.

6   *Very Good*—Does not achieve full swing, timing and coordination consistent.

5   *Good*—Some inconsistency in swing, contact good most of the time. Does not achieve full power.

4   *Average*—Inconsistent in swing and contact, no severe faults.

3   *Fair*—Inconsistent in swing, some faults in form does not maintain body relationship to ball, contact erratic.

2   *Poor*—Several faults in swing, makes contact most of the time but contact seldom produces proper flight.

1   *Very Poor*—Many faults in swing, frequently misses ball, contact usually poor.

NAME	WOODS AND IRONS						
	1	2	3	4	5	6	7
	1	2	3	4	5	6	7
	1	2	3	4	5	6	7

EXAMPLE 7B

PITCH

7 *Excellent*—Size of swing appropriate to distance, consistently produces firm contact, back spin, lofted flight, ball lands within 1 putt distance of cup.

6 *Very Good*—Good swing, sometimes misjudges distance, some loss of accuracy.

5 *Good*—Some inconsistencies in swing, fails to achieve backspin consistently, direction good.

4 *Average*—Inconsistent but can produce a good shot half of the time, distance and direction is erratic.

3 *Fair*—Inconsistent, some faults in form, contact erratic.

2 *Poor*—Several faults in swing, makes contact most of the time but seldom produces proper flight.

1 *Very Poor*—Many faults in swing, contact and flight usually poor.

NAME	PITCH						
	1	2	3	4	5	6	7
	1	2	3	4	5	6	7
	1	2	3	4	5	6	7

Use of Standards

The rating scale presented for the analysis of posture is an example of the use of standards. Photographs or drawings sometimes make the rating more objective and, when there is more than one rater, ratings tend to be more consistent. Use of living models, students chosen from the class to represent various degrees of skill, tends to have a negative effect on those chosen to represent poor skill; and since there are several possible combinations which might represent some of the middle ratings any one model would not represent all of the possibilities.

When the Teacher Is Not the Rater

Most of the discussion thus far has dealt with the type of rating scale which the teacher might use to evaluate his own students. There are circumstances when he might wish to have others make the evaluations and in such cases it may be necessary to include categories which indicate the degree of assurance with which the rater makes the evaluation. Although a rater should have several opportunities to observe, he may still not have had sufficient opportunities to observe

Example 7C
PLAYING DIFFICULT LIES

NAME _____

	Uphill Lies	Downhill Lies	Sidehill Lies	Rough	Sand Trap	Obstacle (bunkers, trees, hills)
Excellent—Chooses appropriate club, ball placed according to lie, stance appropriate to lie, weight and balance maintained throughout stroke, consistent success.	7	7	7	7	7	7
Very Good—Good stroke, does not always choose appropriate club, usually successful.	6	6	6	6	6	6
Good—Some inconsistency in stroke, loses balance occasionally, fairly successful.	5	5	5	5	5	5
Average—Inconsistent in stroke, produces good shot half of the time.	4	4	4	4	4	4
Fair—Inconsistent, some faults in swing, success erratic.	3	3	3	3	3	3
Poor—Several faults, occasional success.	2	2	2	2	2	2
Very Poor—Many faults, usually unsuccessful.	1	1	1	1	1	1

some particular phase for every student. In such a case it is wise to include a space for the rater to check "no opportunity to observe." When several raters' scores are combined into a total score the average score may be assigned to the unobserved rating, or the ratings given may be averaged. For example Jim may have received ratings of 3, 2, 4, and no observation. The mean of the three scores is 3 which could be used as his score, or the mean may be added to the others to give him a total score of 12. Normally a total score is easier to work with than an average; it is easier to arrive at, it involves fewer decimals, and provides a wider range.

EXAMPLE 8

TEAM PLAY

Score	1	2	3	4	5
No opportunity to observe	poor	fair	average	good	excellent

Student Self-Ratings

Having your students rate themselves on their abilities is a useful method of classifying them into groups at the beginning of a unit, or in forming teams when previous evaluation is not possible. Students can also rate themselves on their skills, and this exercise can be a valuable learning experience. The instructor probably would not wish to base his grade on student self-ratings although it has been shown that student self-ratings will correlate as well with instructor ratings as will the average skill test (correlations will fall in the range of .70–.80). Students actually have a rather accurate idea of their capabilities in physical education activity.

Skills Inventory

When planning the program the instructor might wish to assign various amounts of time to different activities, and where possible he might wish to assign students to different activities or to different levels of one activity. A skills inventory, listing the available activities and requesting ability level ratings would provide the necessary information.

This inventory may be analyzed in terms of the needs of the individual student regarding number of skills in which he is intermediate or better, or in which activities he is a beginner. The results may also be analyzed in terms of the activities. If, for instance, the great majority of students are already intermediate or better in basketball, the instructor has an argument for assigning more time to some other activity, or possibly for gearing his instruction to a more advanced level.

Construction of Rating Scales and Check Lists

The steps in the evolution of the check list for the golf swing were as follows:

EXAMPLE 9

NAME _____

CLASS _____

The following list is of activities in which you may now possess some skill. Circle the number most representative of your present skill level.

Activity	Can Not Do	Can Do But Really a Beginner	Would Enter Intermediate Class	Advanced
Archery	0	1	2	3
Badminton	0	1	2	3
Baseball	0	1	2	3
Basketball	0	1	2	3
Folk Dance	0	1	2	3
Golf	0	1	2	3
Gymnastics	0	1	2	3
Soccer	0	1	2	3
Softball	0	1	2	3
Square Dance	0	1	2	3
Swimming	0	1	2	3
Trampoline	0	1	2	3
Track & Field	0	1	2	3
Volleyball	0	1	2	3
Wrestling	0	1	2	3

1. Determine the components of the golf swing.

2. Describe the essentials of each component.

3. Construct a check sheet.

Check sheets are usually designed as class rolls for each component; however, if there are not too many elements, and if descriptions can be kept separate, an individual sheet may be devised containing all elements.

The steps in construction of rating scales are as follows:

1. Determine the elements of the sport.
2. Determine the components of each element.
3. At this point, values are to be assigned, and it is necessary to decide on the number of categories to be used. Possibilities range from three to infinity, although usually not more than 15. Three categories do not allow for much discrimination since they group the students roughly into good, poor, and in the middle; and that can be done without a rating scale. Since most grading systems involve at least five categories (A, B, C, D, F), it might be wise to have at least that many, and since it is sometimes difficult to decide between, say an A or a B, or excellent and not excellent but better than good, you may wish to use seven categories, allowing for more differentiation at the extremes. Some people tend to resist giving the extreme scores, and seven categories still allow for differentiation. The two top and two bottom scores can be combined later to fit into a five-point grading scale. You will note that the examples used are odd numbers; this is to allow for an "average" score, but of course in some situations, average need not be a category. In any case the object is to construct a continuum from one extreme to the other and if possible the steps between intervals should be equal in value, especially if numerical weights are to be assigned which will be added to others to obtain a total score.

EXAMPLE 10

Poor	Fair	Average	Good	Excellent

F	D	C	B	A

4. It is now necessary to describe the categories, and this must be done in terms of a standard. The instructor may wish to use the ideal as his standard, or he may wish his descriptions to be based on the level of his group. An average tennis serve might warrant a different description for a beginner than for a student in an advanced class. Descriptions should be based on the components

found in step (2), as well as in terms of success and consistency. It is usually best to describe in positive terms although there are times when the negative is more helpful.

EXAMPLE 11
TENNIS SERVE

Beginner

5 *Excellent*—Form right in all particulars, consistent, achieves good speed, fairly accurate.

4 *Good*—Good form, lacks speed, is consistent and fairly accurate.

3 *Average*—No severe faults but form could be improved, lacks speed, fairly consistent, gets serve in court.

2 *Fair*—Needs work on most elements of form, inconsistent.

1 *Poor*—Many faults, no speed, inconsistent, inaccurate.

EXAMPLE 12
TENNIS SERVE

Advanced

5 *Excellent*—No faults in form, serve is fast and accurate, consistent.

4 *Good*—No faults in form, good speed, some inconsistency in accuracy.

3 *Average*—Some faults in form, good speed, inconsistent, fairly accurate.

2 *Fair*—Some faults in form, inconsistent, inaccurate, insufficient speed.

1 *Poor*—Several faults in form, inconsistent, inaccurate, poor speed.

5. The final step is to assign numerical values to the rating of each element if scores are to be combined to form a total rating, or to compare a student's ratings on different categories. Once again it is important that the categories be equally spaced in value. Weights may be assigned to different elements according to their importance to the total skill, in which case different weights may be assigned directly to the elements or the element score may be multiplied by the weight value.

Rating Sheets

Several examples of rating sheets have been presented. A class roll may be used with descriptions at the beginning when rating one characteristic as in example 7A; or an individual sheet may be provided for each student as in example 7C. Individual sheets can be

EXAMPLE 13

WOODS AND IRONS (WEIGHT = 3)   SCORE

Very Poor	Poor	Fair	Average	Good	Very Good	Excellent
1	2	3	4	5	6	7

PITCH (WEIGHT = 2)

1	2	3	4	5	6	7

PUTT (WEIGHT = 1)

1	2	3	4	5	6	7

In this example a rating of 4 on each of the skills would receive scores of:

12 (3 × 4) on Woods and Irons
8 (2 × 4) on the Pitch
4 (1 × 4) on Putting

designed to provide a profile when scores on different items can be connected by lines, as in example 14. Weightings may be included and space for the total scores.

EXAMPLE 14

NAME _____

Weight	Serve 2X	Forehand 2X	Backhand 2X	Lob 1X	Smash 1X	Volley 1X	
1						X	
2					X		
3	X		X	X			
4		X					
5							
Weighted Score							TOTAL

Hints on Administration of Rating Scales

Before rating, the instructor should *inform his students* of the purpose of the rating, describe the rating scale, and what they can expect in the rating situation. Unless it is important to the situation that the students be unaware that they are being rated, as might be the case when evaluating the concomitants, the students should be informed so that they will be able to give their best performance, and to avoid the rating situation being too distracting.

The raters should have a *good vantage point* from which to observe the students; however, since some students "clutch" in a pressure situation, if performance under pressure is not a factor in the rating, the pressure can be minimized if it is possible for the rater to observe from a distance.

The raters should have *several opportunities to observe* a performance. This may be achieved by providing for several "attempts" by each student or by rating on more than one occasion, or both. It is also possible to allow a student to try again if he believes that he can improve his score. Once again a student is not tested unless he has, through motivation and the rating situation, the opportunity to do his best.

Normally it is better if the rater can rate one item at a time, for all students. This helps the rater keep the description of exactly what he is rating in his mind and to make comparative judgments if his evaluation is to be made in terms of the group, rather than established criteria.

If the ratings are being made in a competitive situation—game play, for example—then it is best to assure that the competition is between teams or individuals of approximately equal ability. Unequal competition seldom produces good performances.

Of course it is important for the rater to be completely familiar with the rating instrument and know what he is looking for. It is unlikely that a rater would be chosen who is unfamiliar with the activity, but he should be qualified to judge.

Results should be reported and interpreted to the students, and applied to the program according to the purpose for which the ratings were designed.

chapter

4

Administrative Procedures in the Testing Program

There are several steps in the administration of the testing program, careful adherence to which will avoid confusion and insure that the testing will proceed smoothly and the scores be accurate.

Test Selection

The purpose of testing will dictate test selection. Is the evaluation to be of the student or the program? How will the results be used? When the objectives of the testing have been established, the next step is to search for or devise appropriate tests and scrutinize them for their validity and reliability, and their administrative feasibility. A test meeting high statistical standards must also fit within the criteria regarding availability of equipment and facilities, time available for administration, and the instructor's ability to administer the test with the assistants available to him.

Space and Time Planning

Having selected the tests, the next step is to plan for (1) the use of space, (2) the time required to complete each test, and (3) the most efficient organization of the group.

CONSIDERATIONS

1. The first consideration is safety. Sufficient space should be allowed in order to prevent possible injury. An example is the finish line of the shuttle run which should be placed to allow the student to finish at full speed without running into a wall, and if a wall is involved it should be padded. If several tests are to be administered the instructor must make sure that they do not overlap, as with runners crossing into another test area. Pedestrian traffic should be routed around the test area, or the area set up to allow for expected traffic flow and to provide for groups moving from one test area to another.

2. The second consideration is whether or not a test can be administered indoors since some tests require an outdoor space, for example the 50-yard dash and softball throw for distance. Some tests require a floor surface, primarily for safety, as in the obstacle race in the Scott Motor Ability Test; and some tests require a wall or a net. An outside wall may be fine but it must be high enough, and smooth enough; sun and wind might be factors in performance, and the ground surface must be free from hazards. Some tests may be given either outdoors or indoors and can be placed in your plan as space and timing permit.

3. The next consideration is the strenuousness of each test. A student should not be required to take a test when fatigued from a previous test. This may be accomplished by starting with the least strenuous and progressing to the most strenuous tests, or by alternating tests involving different muscle groups or demands on endurance. It would not be wise, for example, to require students to take another test after running the 600.

4. Group organization is the next consideration. There are several choices and which is chosen depends on age level, how much time and how many assistants are available, and the tests themselves.

POSSIBLE GROUP ORGANIZATIONS

A. En masse—When all students are tested at one time, or if partners are needed in the performance of the test half of the group performs at one time while partners assist (e.g., sit-ups).

B. Squads—The group is divided into as many squads as tests, each squad starting at a different test and rotating squads either on signal, or as a squad completes one test it may move to the next area. Tests should consume equal amounts of time for this method to be most effective.

C. Station-to-station—or individual choice. A student rotates as an individual going to each test area without regard to order. This type of organization can be effective with dependable students, previously instructed in the tests and required only to complete each test before finishing.

D. Combinations of above as squads for one or two tests followed by mass for the last test. You might do this on the day you administer the 600-yard run-walk finishing with this event.

5. Timing is the final consideration. Different tests usually require different amounts of time to administer; the size of the group and the time available will determine how many tests can be completed in one session. If the squad method of group organization is to be used multiple stations should be provided for tests requiring more time, in order for the groups to complete the different tests at approximately the same time. It is poor organization to have groups of students waiting too long for the next event. Example 15 provides approximate number of stations needed for equivalent timing for the tests in the AAHPER fitness, and Scott Motor Ability tests.

GYMNASIUM

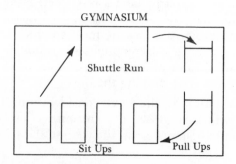

Figure 4.1.

EXAMPLE 15

Number of Stations	
4	Sit-ups (50 maximum)
2	Flex arm hand or pull-ups
2	Broad Jump
2	Basketball Throw (3 throws)
2	Softball Throw (3 throws)
2	Obstacle Race (30 seconds 1 person)
1	Shuttle Run (1 person 2 trials)
1	50-Yard Dash (30 seconds for 2 people)
1	600-Yard Run-Walk (4-5 minutes per group)

40 Students

Period 1 hour   40-45 minutes of activity   AAHPER Fitness Test
Schedule

Monday   3 groups: 2 groups of 14, 1 group of 12

Sit-Ups   4 stations
Pull-Ups   2 stations
Shuttle Run   1 station

Time: 15 minutes per station

Tuesday   **Two groups of 20**

50-yard dash
Broad jump
Softball throw
600-yard Run-Walk

Time: Run 50-yard dash first by twos (10 minutes); two groups of 20, one at broad jump, one at softball throw (20-25 minutes); mass 600-yard run—20 at once, partners score (10 minutes).

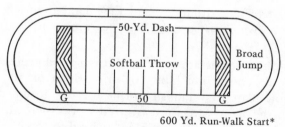

600 Yd. Run-Walk Start*

Figure 4.2.

Note: On a 440 yard track with football field in the middle, begin at back of end zone and run complete circuit and continue to middle of straight (50-yard line).

Note that the indoor tests are set up with appropriate multiple stations to allow each test to be completed in about 15 minutes, although the shuttle run might take slightly less time than the others. In the outdoor tests the 50-yard dash is run first to allow time for recovery before the 600-yard run-walk. The broad jump and softball throw will consume about the same amount of time, and the 600-yard run-walk is kept for last. This is run twice, with each runner having a partner to record his time as he crosses the finish line, after which partners run and first runners record. Should time run out this day, the 600 can be run at the end of the next day's class.

Preparation of Score Cards

TYPE OF SCORE CARD

Score cards may be in the form of class roll sheets, squad cards, or individual score cards. The type of score card used may depend on group organization (mass, squad, individual), the responsibility of the students; i.e., whether they may be depended upon not to lose cards and to record accurately, and the number of tests to be administered (if you are giving only one test, individual score cards would not be needed).

Class rolls are used when only one test is being given or when the instructor needs to make all recordings, as might be the case when testing young children.

Squad cards contain all of the names of the students in a group with spaces provided for recording scores on each test. Squad cards can be used when an assistant at each test station records the scores for a group, and the card is carried from one test area to the next. There is some motivational advantage when scores are readily compared.

Individual score cards have the advantage of involving the student more in the testing situation, and they lend themselves to profile construction, which is an excellent learning and motivation technique.

If established norms are to be used it is a good procedure to either post the scale conversion tables or print them on the score cards. Even if you plan to establish norms for the group, space can be allowed on the score card for converted scores (percentiles, T-scores, etc.) to be entered later. If possible it is good to place conversions on the score cards in such a way to allow scores to be circled and connected into a profile.

Other desired information should be printed on the score cards; such things as name, class, date, age, etc.

EXAMPLE 16

CLASS ROLL OR SQUAD CARD

Name	Sit ups	%	Pull ups	%	Broad Jump	%	S.B. Throw	%	Shuttle Run	%	50-yd Dash	%	600 Run	%	Total	%
John																
Mary																
Sue																
Dave																

EXAMPLE 17

INDIVIDUAL SCORE CARD WITH CONVERSION SCORES

Name _____ Class_____ Date _____

	SCORE	PERCENTILE
Sit-Ups	_____	_____
Pull-Ups	_____	_____
Broad Jump	_____	_____
Shuttle Run	_____	_____
Softball Throw	_____	_____
50-Yard Dash	_____	_____
600-Yard Run	_____	_____

Assistants

If assistants can be trained to help administer the tests the efficiency of the testing program will be increased. If necessary students can help administer the tests, observing results and scoring for each other. In either case assistants need to be instructed and trained in the testing procedures.

EXAMPLE 18
INDIVIDUAL SCORE CARD PROFILE

Name _____ Class _____ Date _____

Percentile	Sit Ups	Pull Ups	Broad Jump	Shuttle Run	SB Throw	50-Yard Dash	600-Yard Run
100	50	40	7'10"	7.5	184	5.4	1:49
95	43	39	6' 6"	10.2	115	7.3	2:19
90	35	38	6' 3"	10.5	103	7.6	2:27
85	31	33	6' 1"	10.7	96	7.7	2:32
80	29	30	5'11"	10.9	90	7.8	2:37
75	27	28	5'10"	11.0	86	7.9	2:41
70	25	26	5' 8"	11.1	82	8.0	2:44
65	24	24	5' 7"	11.2	79	8.1	2:48
60	22	22	5' 6"	11.3	76	8.2	2:51
55	21	21	5' 5"	11.5	73	8.3	2:54
50	20	20	5' 4"	11.6	70	8.4	2:58
45	19	18	5' 3"	11.7	67	8.6	3:01

Instructions

Instructions and demonstrations to be given at each test area should be consistent for each group; it is helpful to write out instructions to be read to the group although it is possible to memorize instructions if they are simple.

Scoring

Scoring should be accurate and results recorded immediately. Usually it is helpful to have an observer (counting, or measuring) and a recorder. When the score to be recorded is the best of several trials it is only necessary to record that best score: for example in the softball throw a scorer can run and stand at the spot of the first throw. If the next throw is longer the first distance need not be held. After the third throw the measurement is made to the point of the longest throw. Only one measurement is made and recorded.

Preparation of the Test Area and Equipment

Make a list of needed supplies, course markings, score cards and pencils, and equipment. Gather materials and mark the course. Sometimes its helpful to identify test stations with signs. When giving two tests requiring one piece of equipment it will be necessary to either have duplicates or not schedule the tests for the same time. If, for example, there are only two stop watches the 50-yard dash and the shuttle run cannot be administered at the same time.

Orient the Students

Before the testing day students should be given instructions regarding dress, scoring and score cards, equipment, groups, rotation, testing procedures, and unless otherwise indicated, practice in the events. Motivation will be increased with discussion of the purpose of the testing and an explanation of how the results will be used.

On the day of the testing, motivation is further increased with encouragement and praise. Safety is best achieved through discipline and pre-instruction, and some warm-up before the testing is advisable to prevent muscle pull.

After Testing

Before the students leave be sure to *collect all score cards.* The next steps are to convert raw scores to scale scores, construct profiles, interpret results, and use the results in the follow-up.

If the instructor is constructing his own norms he will need to find means and standard deviations and convert to standard scores, or find percentiles. Students are usually very interested in testing and are eager to learn how well they performed; results and norms therefore should be presented *as soon as possible.* The student is referred to Chapter 5 for methods of constructing norms.

Since testing is or should be done for some purpose, the results should be used for that purpose: program change, classification of students, or grading.

chapter

5

Statistical Procedures

Having determined our objectives and the importance which we wish to place on each and having selected an appropriate test to administer, having carefully followed directions and collected the scores, we now must handle the data and interpret them. This involves some knowledge of elementary statistics, to the understanding of which we will devote this chapter.

The study of statistical procedures need not be complicated. It does require some use of mathematics and it is understood that many students feel insecure in this area; therefore the student will be taken slowly and carefully through the necessary steps with accompanying discussion of the logic behind each phase. It is not necessary that understanding precede the use of statistics though this is desirable;

for some students understanding is essential while others may achieve results by following the steps and taking their validity on faith.

First let us preview the statistical procedures to be learned and the reasons for learning them.

The first purpose for statistics is to describe either a student's score in terms of the group, or the group itself. For this purpose we need to be able to find the mean, the median, the standard deviation, standard scores, and percentiles.

A second purpose is to compare two groups on some factor, or to check improvement of a group on some factor, or to test one method against another. This requires the standard error of the difference and critical ratio.

A third purpose is to validate a skill test, or to find the relationship between two factors. To do this we find correlation.

There are other procedures necessary to finding some of the items listed but these are essentially the statistical procedures which are presented in this chapter.

Measures of Central Tendency

Susie took the test and scored 67. She asked what that meant and if it was a good score. How did she compare with the others in the class? In the nation? If told that the average score was 50, then her score will be more meaningful—she was better than average. This may not be descriptive enough, but it is a beginning. How is the average score determined?

THE MEAN

First, for the sake of convenience, the student needs to learn some of the symbols associated with statistics. The average score is called the mean. The symbols used in finding the mean are

Σ = sum

X = score

N = number of scores (people)

M = mean (average)

$M = \dfrac{\Sigma X}{N}$

The sum of the scores divided by the number of scores to give you the mean or the average score.

Here is an example of a set of scores, the range of which is from one to ten.

EXAMPLE 19

Score	Frequency		F times Score
10	11	10 X 2 =	20
9	1111	9 X 4 =	36
8	1	8 X 1 =	8
7	1	7 X 1 =	7
6	11	6 X 2 =	12
5	1111	5 X 4 =	20
4	11	4 X 2 =	8
3	11	3 X 2 =	6
2	1	2 X 1 =	2
1	1	1 X 1 =	1
	N = 20		$\Sigma X = 120$

Notice that one person scored 1, one scored 2, two people scored 3, and so on with four scoring 9, and two scoring 10. You could just list the scores individually and add them up to $\Sigma X = 120$. When there are a great many scores however, it is more convenient to tabulate them by frequency of occurrence, and then do some quick multiplication. We have therefore included a frequency column in the form of tally marks. Summing the tallies will provide the number of scores N = 20. The column labled FX is merely composed of each score multiplied by the number of people who made that score, and the sum of the column provides $\Sigma X = 120$. We now have all of the information necessary to find the mean. In this case $M = \dfrac{\Sigma X}{N} = \dfrac{120}{20} = 6$. The average score on this distribution is 6.

PROBLEM 1

Find the mean of the following distribution:

Score		
X	F	FX
10	1	
9	111	
8	⊞⊞⊞	
7	1111	
6	⊞⊞⊞	
5	⊞⊞⊞	
4	11	
3	111	
2	1	
1	1	
	N = _____	$\Sigma X =$ _____

$$M = \frac{\Sigma X}{N} = \underline{\hspace{1cm}}$$

THE MEDIAN

Although the mean is the most used measure of central tendency there is another measure which is useful in certain cases, for example in a bowling class in which averages are kept. Suppose we had two students averaging 150 while the scores of the rest of the class, truly beginners, ranged about 90. The 150 averages when added to the other scores would raise the mean of the group above the score which was most representative of the class. This would be especially true if it were a small class. In a case such as this the median would be a truer indication of central tendency. The median is the score above which are half of the class and below which are half of the class, the 50th percentile. To find the median we divide N by 2 and count up or down until we reach half of the group. In the case of Example 19 the median falls between 5 and 6 with 10 people above and 10 people below. The median is 5.5, halfway between 5 and 6.

A number occupies a space; the number 5 occupies a space from 4.5 to 5.5.

3.5	4	4.5	5	5.5	6	6.5

If our count, as in Example 19, ends at the top of the number 5 then the median is 5.5. Should our count end in a number occupied by several people, $\begin{array}{cc} X & f \\ 5 & 1111 \end{array}$, with the halfway point falling one person into the four people scoring 5 then we take that fraction (¼) of the number and add it to the bottom of the number if we are counting up, or subtract it from the top if we are counting down. In this case we would add ¼ or .25 to 4.5 (the bottom of number 5) and the median would be 4.75. If three people occupy the number then we add thirds. If an odd number such as seven is involved we divide 7 into the number 1.00 to find 1/7th, and multiply the result by the number of people needed to reach the mid point.

THE MODE

A third indication of central tendency is the mode. This is the score most frequently made, and it is possible to have more than one mode as in example 19. The modes are 5 and 9. What is the mode in

Problem 2? _____

PROBLEM 2

Find the median on the following distributions:

Score	
X	F
10	11
9	1111
8	1111
7	111
6	~~1111~~ 11
5	1111
4	11
3	11
2	1
1	1
	N = 30

Median = _____

PROBLEM 3

If counting up from the bottom (zero) the half-way tally fell two people into five people occupying the number 8, what would be the Median? _____

The Normal Curve

The mean is most useful when the distribution is normal, for as we have seen a distribution which has exceptional scores at an extreme will yield a distorted mean. Most statistical procedures are based on the assumption that the scores assume a normal distribution, or that they would do so if N were large. The two bowlers who averaged 150 would affect the mean greatly if there were only 10 members in the class, and not nearly so much if they were only two of one hundred scores. The student is familiar with grading systems based on "the curve." The curve is the normal probability curve, based on the likelihood of scores occurring by chance.

The normal curve based on probability looks as that in Figure 5.1, with the mean at the highest point. In a normal distribution the mean, median, and mode all occupy the same score.

The student will note the divisions around the mean. These are standard deviations which will enclose certain percentages of scores. For example, in the area under the curve enclosed by one standard

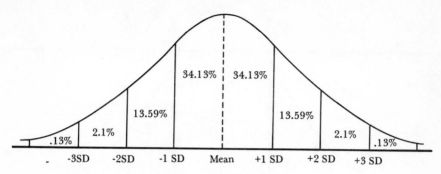

Figure 5.1. The Normal Curve.

deviation above and one SD below the mean there will be found almost 70 percent of the scores (34.13 percent + 34.13 percent = 68.26 percent). The area enclosed by two standard deviations above and below the mean includes approximately 95 percent of the scores (13.59 percent + 34.13 percent + 34.13 percent + 13.59 percent = 95.44 percent).

The Standard Deviation—A Measure of Variability

The standard deviation (SD) is a measure of the spread of scores around the mean. A small SD ("small" is relative to the scores which we are using, for example, a SD of 10 on a distribution of 100 is equivalent to a SD of 1 on a distribution of 10) indicates that the scores cluster around the mean. A large SD indicates that the scores are spread widely. See figure 5.2.

The student who scored 67 on the test with a mean of 50 had a deviation score of +17. He was 17 points above the mean. A student with a 52 would have a deviation score of +2, and a score of 45 would yield a deviation score of -5.

If the SD of a distribution were known then it would be possible to determine the percentage of scores above and below any one score. Now our student's 67 can be placed, not only above the mean, but how far above the mean and how many scores are above him.

For example, if the mean were 50 and the SD 10 then a 67 would be 1.7 standard deviations above the mean. This is found by subtracting the mean from the score (67 - 50) and dividing by the SD (17 ÷ 10 = 1.7). The student is 1.7 standard deviations above the mean. This is his standard score.

Table 5.1 provides the areas under the normal curve and can be read as follows on page 207.

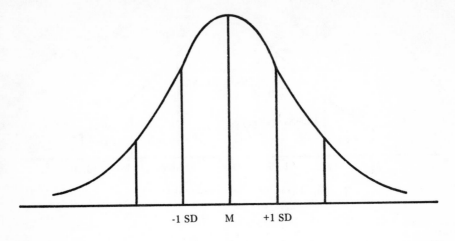

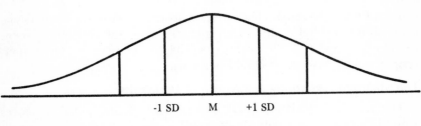

Figure 5.2.

The column labelled units is the deviation score divided by the standard deviation. This column gives the whole number and one decimal. The next columns labelled .00, .01, etc., give the second decimal. In our example a score of 67 yielded a standard score of 1.70. Finding 1.7 in the first column we read for the second decimal (zero in this case) and find the figure 45.54. This figure represents a percentage of 45.54 above the mean. Since 50 percent of the scores are below the mean a score of 67 in this instance would fall at the point at which 95.54 percent (50 + 45.54) of the scores are below it, and our student is in the upper 5 percent of the class.

CALCULATION OF THE STANDARD DEVIATION

When we subtracted the score from the mean, we were finding the student's deviation score—how he deviated from the mean. With a mean of 50 a score of 52 would have a deviation score of +2, a score

Table 5.1

Percentage Parts of the Total Area under the Normal Probability Curve Corresponding to Distances on the Base Line between the Mean and Successive Points from the Mean in Units of Standard Deviation.*

Example: Between the mean and a point 1.57 sigma is found 44.18 per cent of the entire area under the curve.

Units	.00	.01	.02	.03	.04	.05	.06	.07	.08	.09
0.0	00.00	00.40	00.80	01.20	01.60	01.99	02.39	02.79	03.19	03.59
0.1	03.98	04.38	04.78	05.17	05.57	05.96	06.36	06.75	07.14	07.53
0.2	07.93	08.32	08.71	09.10	09.48	09.87	10.26	10.64	11.03	11.41
0.3	11.79	12.17	12.55	12.93	13.31	13.68	14.06	14.43	14.80	15.17
0.4	15.54	15.91	16.28	16.64	17.00	17.36	17.72	18.08	18.44	18.79
0.5	19.15	19.50	19.85	20.19	20.54	20.88	21.23	21.57	21.90	22.24
0.6	22.57	22.91	23.24	23.57	23.89	24.22	24.54	24.86	25.17	25.49
0.7	25.80	26.11	26.42	26.73	27.04	27.34	27.64	27.94	28.23	28.52
0.8	28.81	29.10	29.39	29.67	29.95	30.23	30.51	30.78	31.06	31.33
0.9	31.59	31.86	32.12	32.38	32.64	32.90	33.15	33.40	33.65	33.89
1.0	34.13	34.38	34.61	34.85	35.08	35.31	35.54	35.77	35.99	36.21
1.1	36.43	36.65	36.86	37.08	37.29	37.49	37.70	37.90	38.10	38.30
1.2	38.49	38.69	38.88	39.07	39.25	39.44	39.62	39.80	39.97	40.15
1.3	40.32	40.49	40.66	40.82	40.99	41.15	41.31	41.47	41.62	41.77
1.4	41.92	42.07	42.22	42.36	42.51	42.65	42.79	42.92	43.06	43.19
1.5	43.32	43.45	43.57	43.70	43.83	43.94	44.06	44.18	44.29	44.41
1.6	44.52	44.63	44.74	44.84	44.95	45.05	45.15	45.25	45.35	45.45
1.7	45.54	45.64	45.73	45.82	45.91	45.99	46.08	46.16	46.25	46.33
1.8	46.41	46.49	46.56	46.64	46.71	46.78	46.86	46.93	46.99	47.06
1.9	47.13	47.19	47.26	47.32	47.38	47.44	47.50	47.56	47.61	47.67
2.0	47.72	47.78	47.83	47.88	47.93	47.98	48.03	48.08	48.12	48.17
2.1	48.21	48.26	48.30	48.34	48.38	48.42	48.46	48.50	48.54	48.57
2.2	48.61	48.64	48.68	48.71	48.75	48.78	48.81	48.84	48.87	48.90
2.3	48.93	48.96	48.98	49.01	49.04	49.06	49.09	49.11	49.13	49.16
2.4	49.18	49.20	49.22	49.25	49.27	49.29	49.31	49.32	49.34	49.36
2.5	49.38	49.40	49.41	49.43	49.45	49.46	49.48	49.49	49.51	49.52
2.6	49.53	49.55	49.56	49.57	49.59	49.60	49.61	49.62	49.63	49.64
2.7	49.65	49.66	49.67	49.68	49.69	49.70	49.71	49.72	49.73	49.74
2.8	49.74	49.75	49.76	49.77	49.77	49.78	49.79	49.79	49.80	49.81
2.9	49.81	49.82	49.82	49.83	49.84	49.84	49.85	49.85	49.86	49.86
3.0	49.865									
3.1	49.903									
3.2	49.93129									
3.3	49.95166									
3.4	49.96631									
3.5	49.97674									
3.6	49.98409									
3.7	49.98922									
3.8	49.99277									
3.9	49.99519									

*Adapted from: *Biometrika Tables for Statisticians,* Vol. 1, 1954, Edited by E.S. Pearson and H.O. Hartley, Located in Mathews, Donald K., *Measurement in Physical Education.* Third edition, Philadelphia: W.B. Saunders Co., 1963. Used by permission of the publisher.

PROBLEM 4

Find the percentage of scores below the following

$$M = 50$$
$$SD = 10$$
$$\text{Score I} = 60$$

a. deviation score =

b. standard score =

c. percent scores between M and standard score =

$$50 + c =$$

Score II = 45

a. deviation score =

b. standard score =

c. percent scores between M and standard score =

$$50 - c =$$

Note: 45 is below the mean therefore he is in the lower 50 percent of scores and the
percent of scores between his score and the mean must be subtracted from the mean
to find the percentage below him.

of 70, +20; 40, -10; 23, -27; etc. It is possible to find the standard
deviation using the original scores but numbers frequently get quite
large and it is usually more convenient to work with deviation scores
(d) which are smaller. The formula for standard deviation is $\sqrt{\dfrac{\Sigma d^2}{N}}$.
Example 20 shows how to calculate the standard deviation.

In this example we have already found the mean to be 6 (the
student may wish to practice on this distribution by including the
FX column and finding the mean).

Since the mean is 6, a score of six does not deviate from it and
therefore receives a deviation score of zero. Each step up or down
from the mean receives either a positive or negative deviation score,
as a score of 7 would be +1, and a score of 5 equals a deviation score
of -1.

Our next step is to square each of the deviation scores; this column is labelled d^2. Squaring a number exaggerates its largeness or
smallness; for example: 1 squared is still 1, while 5 squared leaps to
25. This exaggeration serves to emphasize the distribution around the
mean and tends to make the standard deviation more useful. For the
5th column labelled $f(d)^2$ we multiply each d^2 by the number of

EXAMPLE 20

STANDARD DEVIATION
Deviation Scores

X	F	$(X-M) = d*$	d^2	$f(d^2)$
10	1	$10 - 6 = 4$	16	16
9	1	$9 - 6 = 3$	9	9
8	2	$9 - 6 = 2$	4	8
7	3	$7 - 6 = 1$	1	3
M = 6	6	$6 - 6 = 0$	0	0
5	3	$5 - 6 = -1$	1	3
4	2	$4 - 6 = -2$	4	8
3	1	$3 - 6 = -3$	9	9
2	1	$2 - 6 = -4$	16	16
1	0	$1 - 6 = -5$	25	0
	N = 20			$\Sigma d^2 = 72$

$$SD = \sqrt{\frac{\Sigma d^2}{N}}$$

$$SD = \sqrt{\frac{72}{20}} = \sqrt{3.6}$$

$$SD = 1.9$$

```
    1.  9
  ⌈3.  60
    1
29 ⌈260
    261
```

*$d = X - M$ (e.g., $9 - 6 = 3$ and $2 - 6 = -4$)

people holding that score (f) as we did in finding the mean. For example: two people scored 8, the deviation score for 8 is +2, and 2 squared is 4. Two 4's give us 8 in this column. Note that no one scored a 1 and therefore 5 deviations below the mean multiplied by zero gives us a zero.

When summed, column 5 provides Σd^2 which is put in the formula for standard deviation, and is divided by N (20). Since we squared earlier, and since have completed the function we need now to un-square, to bring the figures back to their original context.

FINDING THE SQUARE ROOT

It might be helpful here to review a method of taking a square root. We may of course refer to a table of squares; however, there are times when one is working with fractional numbers that it is more convenient to work the problem by hand. The following steps will solve the problem.

EXAMPLE I   **EXAMPLE II**

$$\sqrt{21.\,00\,00}$$

1. Set up your numbers in groups of two on either side of the decimal moving away from the decimal.

$$\sqrt{01\,81.\,72\,00}$$

$$\overset{4}{\sqrt{21.\,00\,00}}$$

2. Find the largest number which when squared will go into the first group on the left and place it above the group.

$$\overset{1}{\sqrt{01\,81.\,72\,00}}$$

$$\begin{array}{r} 4 \\ \sqrt{21.\,00\,00} \\ 16 \\ \hline 5\,00 \end{array}$$

3. Square that number and subtract it from group 1, and bring down the next group.

$$\begin{array}{r} 1 \\ \sqrt{01\,81.\,72\,00} \\ 1 \\ \hline 81 \end{array}$$

$$8\quad\begin{array}{r} 4 \\ \sqrt{21.\,00\,00} \\ 16 \\ \hline 5\,00 \end{array}$$

4. Multiply the top number by 2 and place it in the division position allowing space for a second digit.

$$2\quad\begin{array}{r} 1 \\ \sqrt{01\,81.\,72\,00} \\ 1 \\ \hline 81 \end{array}$$

$$85\quad\begin{array}{r} 4.\ 5 \\ \sqrt{21.\,00\,00} \\ 16 \\ \hline 5\,00 \\ 4\,25 \\ \hline 75 \end{array}$$

5. Estimate the number, which at this point will be a two digit number, which will divide into your dividend, and place the second digit in the divisor *and* above the second group.

$$23\quad\begin{array}{r} 1\ 3. \\ \sqrt{01\,81.\,72\,00} \\ 1 \\ \hline 81 \\ 69 \\ \hline 12 \end{array}$$

$$\begin{array}{r} 4.\ 5\ 8\ 2 \\ \sqrt{21.\,00\,00\,00} \\ 16 \end{array}$$

$$85\quad\begin{array}{r} 5\,00 \\ 4\,25 \end{array}$$

$$908\quad\begin{array}{r} 75\,00 \\ 72\,64 \end{array}$$

6. Multiply the new divisor by the last chosen digit and subtract the result from the dividend.

$$9162\quad\begin{array}{r} 2\,36\,00 \\ 1\,83\,24 \\ \hline 52\,76 \end{array}$$

Answer = 4.58

$$\begin{array}{r} 1\ 3.\ 4\ 8\ 0 \\ \sqrt{01\,81.\,72\,00\,00} \\ 1 \end{array}$$

$$23\quad\begin{array}{r} 0\,81 \\ 69 \end{array}$$

$$264\quad\begin{array}{r} 12\,72 \\ 10\,56 \end{array}$$

$$2688\quad\begin{array}{r} 2\,16\,00 \\ 2\,15\,04 \end{array}$$

$$2696\quad\quad 96\,00$$

Answer = 13.48

7. Repeat steps 4—6 with the new number.

Carry the square root to three decimals and round back to two decimals. Calculations may be checked by squaring the result.

Problem 5

Find the SD for the following scores:

X	F	FX	d	d^2	$f(d^2)$
20	1				
19	1				
18	1				
17	11				
16	11				
15	0				
14	0				
13	111				
12	11				
11	111				
10	~~1111~~ 1				
9	1111				
8	111				
7	111				
6	111				
5	0				
4	11				
3	11				
2	1				
1	1				

N = _____ ΣX = ____ Σd^2 _____ $M = \dfrac{\Sigma X}{N}$ =

$$SD = \sqrt{\frac{\Sigma d^2}{N}} = \underline{\hspace{3cm}}$$

Standard Scores and Percentiles

When we divided one student's deviation score by the SD of the distribution we in effect changed it into another form, the number of SD's it was from the mean. This is the same process we use when we convert inches to feet, we divide by the unit for feet (12 inches). In this case we convert a score into standard scores. Standard scores are always comparable no matter what units we are using, whether they be inches, seconds, centimeters, or just numbers; when they are reported as standard scores the student can be placed in an equivalent position on all of his tests.

For example, he may have the following scores on the broad jump, 50-yard dash, and a rules test; means, SD's, and standard scores are given:

EXAMPLE 21

	X	M	SD	d/SD
Broad Jump	6'1"	5'10"	6"	+3"/6" = +0.5
50-Yard Dash	5 sec.	7 sec.	1 sec.	+2 /1 = +2.0
Rules Test	80	50	12	+30/12 = +2.5

On the normal curve his positions in the three tests would fall as pictured in Figure 5.3.

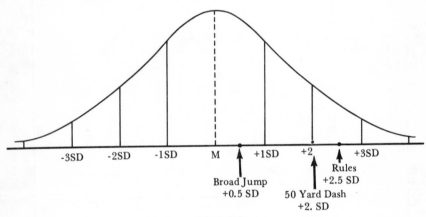

Figure 5.3.

The student might like to find the percentage of scores below his score by referring to Table 5.1.

Of course standard scores are meaningful, but we are accustomed to thinking of scores in terms of a hundred point scale and there are three commonly used methods of converting standard scores to 100 point scales. We shall learn to use each, for each has an advantage and a disadvantage.

SIGMA, HULL, AND T SCALES

Once again we return to the normal curve, but now where our range of scores might have been 3 to 10 seconds, 4 to 7 feet, or 10 to 90 points each will be converted to points ranging from 0 to 100.

Figure 5.4 depicts the conversion scales for the Sigma, Hull and T scores. Note that the mean is always 50 and the SD's are spaced equally with our original distribution. The size of the SD's of each scale will vary with the number of SD's incorporated between zero and 100. The Sigma scale encompasses 6 SD's between 0 and 100, the Hull scale uses 7 SD's, 3 1/2 above and 3 1/2 below the mean, while the T scale uses 10 SD's.

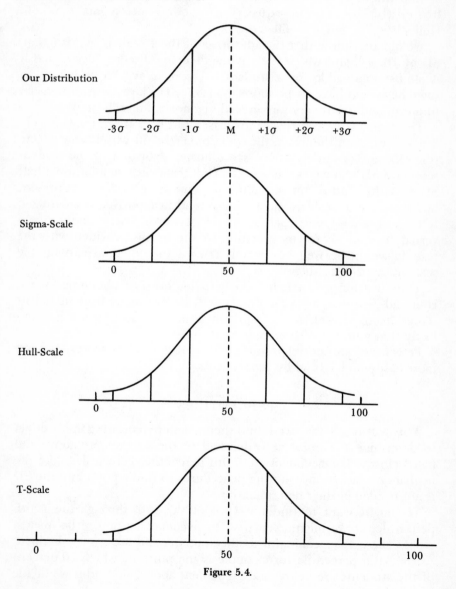

Figure 5.4.

In order to know how large the SD is in each, you need only divide 100 points by the number of SD's involved; therefore the SD of the Sigma scale is $100 \div 6 = 16.66$ points. The Hull SD is $100 \div 7 = 14.29$ points, and the SD for the T scale is $100 \div 10 = 10$. This is the advantage of the T scale. The mean is always 50 with an SD of 10 and easily handled.

Knowing this, if a student scored 1 SD above the mean on a test he could be given equivalent scores of: Sigma = 66.66, Hull = 64.29, and T = 60.

We already know that the advantage of the T scale is that it has an SD of 10, a figure which is easily handled; its disadvantage is that it is almost impossible for a student to score above 85 or below 15 since he would have to be more than 3.5 SD's away from the mean to do so, and this is very rare indeed in a normal distribution.

The Sigma scale will cover most cases, but because its range is only 3 SD's out from the mean, the occasional student who is very exceptional is not rewarded with a score higher than that of the student scoring 3 SD's above the mean. The Hull scale with an additional half SD on either end of the distribution seems more realistic. At present however, the T scale is most widely used in reporting standardized tests, and when giving such a test our students' scores may be converted to scale scores by referring to the norms provided with the test. It would be well however if the instructor could explain the scale scores to his student.

Your instructor can help you with methods of obtaining Sigma, Hull and T scores; however since you will not usually have sufficient scores from your classes to represent a normal distribution it is unlikely that you will wish to convert them to these scales.

Percentiles are more appropriately used with class scores, and are more easily understood by the students.

PERCENTILES

You will recall that we found the median by counting up or down to determine the point at which half of the scores were above and half below. The median is the 50th percentile. Percentiles, like the median are based on counting procedures to find a point and the SD is not needed in their determination.

We might want to find the 10th, 20th, 30th through the 100th percentile, or we might even wish to give an exact percentile to each score. These are meaningful to the students and are easily obtained.

The 10th percentile for example is the point at which 10 percent of the students are below and 90 percent above. To find it we divide the number of scores (people) by ten, count up from the bottom (lowest score) until we pass that number and figure the percentile point as we did the median.

If we had 100 students, then each student would be 1 percent of our group, and each percentile could be figured for each student. Normally it is sufficient to figure percentiles in groups of 10.

If for example we had 40 students, then dividing 40 by 10 (ten percentiles) we would count up 4 people to determine each 10th percentile.

EXAMPLE 22

	X	f	cf	Percentile score	Percentile
100th	10	1	40	10.0	P 100
90th	9	11	39	8.25	P 90
80th	8	111 1	37	7.30	P 80
70th	7	1111 1	33	6.50	P 70
60th	6	111 1111	28	5.93	P 60
50th	5	111 1111 1	21	5.37	P 50
40th	4	1111 1	13	4.87	P 40
30th	3	1111	8	4.30	P 30
20th	2	111	4	3.50	P 20
10th	1	1	1	2.50	P 10
				1.00	P 0

N = 40

The cf column is the cumulated frequencies added from the bottom. Note that counting 4 people from the bottom of the distribution brings us to the end of score number 2, and you will recall that the number 2 occupies the space 1.5—2.5; therefore the 10th percentile (P 10) is at the top of the number 2 (2.5). Four more people bring us to the top of score number 3 (3.5), and four more brings us 4/5 of the way through the number 4. Four fifths of 1.00 is .80 (1.00 ÷ 5 = .20, 4 × .20 = 80) and .80 added to the bottom of number 4 (3.5) is 4.3 (3.50 + .80 = 4.30). The process continues to P 100. P 100 is *always* the highest score achieved, and P 0 is always the lowest score achieved.

The next step is to round the percentile scores. In our example the range of scores is not great enough to prevent duplication of percentiles in one score. Example 23 depicts a wider range of scores; however even this range presents some problems.

EXAMPLE 23

X	f	Percentile Score	Rounded	Percentile
20	1	20.4	20	P 100
19	1			
18	1			
17	1 1	17.0	17	P 90
16	11			
15				
14				
13	11 1	13.16	13	P 80
12	11			
11	111	11.50	12	P 70
10	1 1111 1	10.35	11	P 60
9	1 111	9.67	10	P 50
8	111	8.75	9	P 40
7	111	7.50	8	P 30
6	11 1	6.17	6	P 20
5				
4	11			
3	11	3.50	4	P 10
2	1			
1	1	1.00	1	P 0
	N = 40			

In this example we can see the complications which can arise in determining placement of the percentiles. P 10, P 20, P 30, and P 40 are fairly simple and we can designate the whole number involved as that representing the percentile. When we reach score number 10 we find two percentile groups falling in one score (P 50, P 60); however since the score 11 is not occupied and 9 is occupied we may designate 11 as P 60.

These data may now be interpreted as follows: For example a student scoring 12 is in the upper 30 percent of the group—the 70th percentile, while a score of 6 places him in the 20th percentile with approximately 80 percent of the class scoring better than he.

Reliability of the Mean

When the instructor gives a test to his class the resulting scores, mean, and SD describe his group. His students are a sample group of a population; for example a senior boy in a volleyball class is a part of all senior boys in the school, in the town, in the state, country, and even in the world. Each sub-group is a sample of the larger group, presumably a representative sample, typical senior high boys.

PROBLEM 6

Find the percentile scores for P 10, P 50, and P 80 for the following distribution:

X	f	
		P 80 = _____
10	1	
9	11	
8	1111	
7	11111	
6	11111 11	P 50 = _____
5	11111 111	
4	11111	
3	1111	P 10 = _____
2	111	
1	1	

The question to be asked then is, are the scores obtained in the class typical of scores which would be obtained if we measured all senior boys on the same test?

As we noted earlier when finding the median, one or two scores can affect the mean considerably, especially if the group is small. Our example was a bowling class in which most students averaged around 90 while two students averaged 150. Suppose the class size were twelve students, ten of whom average 90, and two with averages of 150. The mean would be roughly:

$$10 \times 90 = 900$$
$$2 \times 150 = \underline{300}$$
$$\Sigma X = \overline{1200}$$
$$M = \frac{\Sigma X}{N} = \frac{1200}{12} = 100$$

The two high-scoring students have raised the mean of the rest of the class 10 points.

Should we, instead, have 100 students, 98 averaging 90 and two averaging 150 our mean would be:

$$98 \times 90 = 8820$$
$$2 \times 150 = \underline{300}$$
$$\Sigma X = \overline{9120}$$
$$M = \frac{\Sigma X}{N} = \frac{9120}{100} = 91.2$$

This time the two 150 averages have raised the mean only 1.2 point. They still affect the mean but not nearly as much when N is large.

In any sample one score will affect the mean, and if the sample is small the mean may be greatly affected; if the spread of scores is large, as 60-150 compared with 80-110, then the scores at the extremes will exert a greater influence on the mean than they would with a small range of scores.

THE STANDARD ERROR OF THE MEAN (SE$_m$)

In order to judge how far our sample mean might be from the population mean (that mean we would obtain if we tested every senior boy) we need to find the standard error of the mean.

The standard error of the mean is a function of

1. The number of cases (N)
2. The variability or spread of the scores (SD)

The addition of one score will change the mean; and the smaller the number of cases the greater will be the effect of that one score on the mean. (Actually reliability increases in proportion to the square root of N rather than N itself.)

If the SD of the distribution is small we may assume that the true mean falls close to the obtained mean, because the majority of the scores fall within + or - one SD; therefore as SD decreases the reliability of the mean increases.

The formula for the standard error of the mean (SE_m) is $\frac{SD}{\sqrt{N}}$. The student can see that this formula makes maximum use of SD and N, and that as SD gets smaller and N larger the SE$_m$ will be smaller.

The means of many sample groups such as ours would tend to form a distribution of their own, and this distribution would fall on the pattern of the normal probability curve, with the hypothetical true mean as its mean. The SE of the mean is in effect the SD of this distribution of possible sample means.

Figure 5.5 depicts the hypothetical distribution of sample means, with a possible position of our sample mean in relation to the true mean.

As an example: If we had 50 physical education majors with a mean of 20.0 (on the obstacle race) and a SD of 1.75, the SE$_m$ would be

$$\frac{1.75}{\sqrt{50}} \quad = \quad \frac{1.75}{7.07} \quad = \quad 2.47 \text{ or } .25.$$

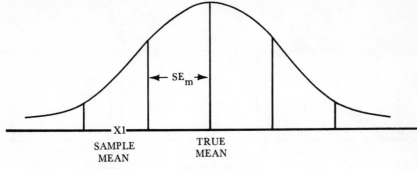

Figure 5.5.

PROBLEM 7

Find the standard error of the mean for the following:

$$M = 60$$
$$N = 25$$
$$SD = 5$$

$$SE_m = \frac{SD}{\sqrt{N}} = \underline{\hspace{4cm}}$$

Significance of the Difference Between Means

Thus far we have learned to describe one group by the measures of central tendency (M, Med.), measure of distribution (SD), and measure of the reliability of our mean (SE_m). When we wish to compare performances of two groups we look at the difference (D) between the means $D = (M_1 - M_2)$. We must now wonder whether this difference is a true difference or a product of chance.

In Figure 5.6 we show the distribution of sample means with two sample means falling at the extremes of the distribution. Note the size of the difference which could result from two sample means and yet that difference still be only the result of sampling error.

THE STANDARD ERROR OF THE DIFFERENCE BETWEEN MEANS (SE$_D$)

In order to discover whether the two groups differ significantly we need a standard error of the difference between the means. The

formula for SE$_D$ is: $\quad \sqrt{SE_{m_1}^{\,2} + SE_{m_2}^{\,2}}$

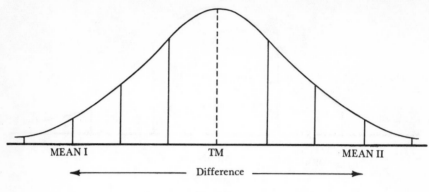

MEAN I   TM   MEAN II

◄─────────────── Difference ───────────────►

Figure 5.6.

In essence we have added the standard errors of the two means. We have however squared them before adding, and then taken the square root, since this allows very small or very large SE_m's to have a greater influence on the SE_D, and this is as it should be.

The SE_D is actually the measure of the spread of a distribution of all possible sample differences if we set the true difference at zero. We are starting with the assumption that the actual difference between the groups is zero and we want to find out whether or not our obtained difference (D) could have happened by chance sampling fluctuations.

It can be seen that if we collected a number of sample means, differences would exist between them. Actually we could obtain a great number of differences for if we compare each mean with each other mean we would have $\frac{N(N-1)}{2}$ differences.

In this formula N represents the number of sample means obtained; (N - 1) represents the number of comparisons to be made for each mean. Each mean will be compared with every other mean (one less than N since it won't be compared with itself). We divide by two because when mean A is compared with mean B the difference is the same as a comparison of mean B with mean A.

In Figure 5.7 we see the hypothetical distribution of possible differences which we might obtain from any two samples. While the true difference is really zero, the measure of dispersion is the standard error of the differences (SE_D).

EXAMPLE 24

Suppose we have collected ten sample means. The number of differences we would get would be $\dfrac{10 \times 9}{2} = 45$.

These 45 differences would form a distribution of their own. Should we collect 10,000 sample means we would have

$$\frac{10,000 \times 9,999}{2} = 49,995,000$$

differences. Of course many of the differences would be the same and our distribution would assume the shape of the normal probability curve.

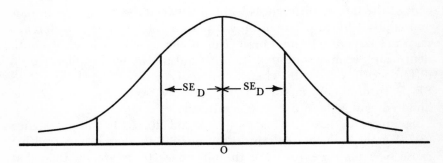

Figure 5.7

PROBLEM 8

Find the SE_D for the following:

$$SE_{m_1} = 4$$
$$SE_{m_2} = 3$$
$$SE_D = \sqrt{SE_{m_1}^2 + SE_{m_2}^2}$$

$$SE_D = \underline{\hspace{3cm}}$$

The Critical Ratio (t)

When we studied the normal curve we found we could determine the percentage of scores between the mean and any standard deviation or fraction thereof. Table 5.1 indicates that 95 percent of the scores fall between the mean plus and minus 1.96 SD's, and that 99 percent of the scores fall between the mean plus and minus 2.58 SD's. These are crucial points in determining whether a difference occurred from sampling error, or whether there really was a real difference between the groups. In this case 95 percent of the possible sampling differences will fall between mean plus 1.96 SE_D's and mean minus 1.96 SE_D's, and similarly 99 percent of sample differences will fall between mean plus and minus 2.58 SE_D's.

These critical points are called levels of confidence, for if 95 percent of the sample differences will fall between the mean of zero plus and minus 1.96 SE_D's then only 5 percent of the sample difference may fall outside of this range. This is the 5 percent level of confidence, and we may state that 95 times out of 100 we would *not* get a difference this large by chance. Similarly a difference falling 2.58 SE_D's from the mean of zero could only occur one time in one hundred, and is therefore very significant.

Suppose we have means of 24.45 and 20.66. Is this difference (3.79) great enough to exclude the possibility that it occurred because of sampling error? For the difference to be greater than that allowed by sampling error it must be beyond the curve of possible chance differences when the true difference is zero. Therefore it must be greater than 1.96 or 2.58 SE_D's from the mean of zero.

In order to change our difference into SE_D's we divide it by the SE_D and obtain the critical ratio, $t = D/SE_D$. The critical ratio is the number of SE_D's our difference is from the mean of zero. (Note: CR is usually indicated by t in research literature.)

In our example with D = 3.79

$$SE_D = .60$$

$$t = \frac{D}{SE_D} = \frac{3.79}{0.60} = 6.32$$

In our example the CR was 6.32 which would place our difference 6.32 SE_D's from the mean of zero; certainly well beyond the possibility of chance and therefore very significant. See Figure 5.8.

If our CR is small, say .79 then we must say that our difference could very well have been due to sampling differences and we cannot honestly say the difference is significant.

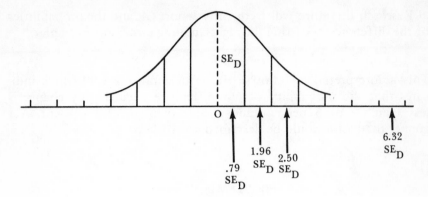

Figure 5.8

EXAMPLE 25
OBSTACLE RACE

Freshmen P.E. Majors		Sophomore and Junior P.E. Majors	
M	22.15	M	20.66
SD	2.22	SD	1.75
N	54	N	44

$$SE_D = \sqrt{\frac{(2.22)^2}{54} + \frac{(1.75)^2}{44}}$$

$$SE_D = \sqrt{.091 + .069} = \sqrt{.16}$$

$$SE_D = .4$$

$$D = 22.15 - 20.66$$

$$D = 1.49$$

$$t = \frac{1.49}{.40} = 3.72$$

Our significance levels are:

   .05 = 1.96

   .01 = 2.58

Since our obtained CR is greater than either of these we may say that the difference is significant at the .01 (1%) level of confidence.

Note that it is not necessary to find SE_m since $SE_m{}^2 = \left(\frac{SD}{\sqrt{N}}\right)^2 = \frac{SD^2}{N}$ which is placed

directly under the square root in the formula for SE_D.

Research literature will frequently report CR and the probabilities of the difference occurring through sampling error. For example:

$$t = 1.98 \qquad\qquad .05 > p > .01$$

This is interpreted as follows: the critical ratio is 1.98 which indicates that the probability of our difference occurring by chance is less than ($> p$) 5 percent and greater than ($p >$) 1 percent. A t greater than 2.58 would be described as: $.01 > p$.

PROBLEM 9

Find the critical ratio for the following:

Group I			Group II		
M_1	=	35	M_2	=	41
SD_1	=	5	SD_1	=	4
N_1	=	25	N_1	=	49

$$SE_{m_1} = \frac{SD_1}{\sqrt{N}} = \rule{2cm}{0.4pt} \qquad SE_{m_2} = \frac{SD_2}{\sqrt{N}} = \rule{2cm}{0.4pt}$$

$$SE_D = \sqrt{SE_{m_1}^{\,2} + SE_{m_2}^{\,2}} = \rule{2cm}{0.4pt} \qquad \text{Alternate formula for } SE_D$$

$$D = M_1 - M_2 = \rule{2cm}{0.4pt}$$

$$t = \frac{D}{SE_D} = \rule{2cm}{0.4pt} \qquad\qquad \sqrt{\frac{SD_1^{\,2}}{N_1} + \frac{SD_2^{\,2}}{N_2}}$$

Correlation

When we were thinking of test selection we found it necessary to consider validity and reliability. These qualities are reported in terms of coefficients of correlation (r), and we found that these range from -1.00 to +1.00. The student might wish to review the discussion on correlation in Chapter 2.

We have since learned to compare the differences between the means of two different groups. When we want to compare the same group on two different tests, or on the same test given twice (before and after for example), then we need to consider the amount of correlation existing between the two sets of scores.

The coefficient of correlation is a ratio which indicates the amount of relationship existing between two sets of scores. For example, we would expect a relationship to exist between a student's height and the height of the highest point which he could touch on the jump reach test. If we correlated these two measures (height and jump height), we would get considerable agreement.

Assuming height to be the only factor in this test,* we would expect the tallest student to touch the highest point; the second tallest, the second highest point; and so on to the shortest student and the lowest point. If this were true, we would get a perfect correlation. Actually we won't get this result for frequently a shorter student will be able to out-jump a taller student and touch a higher mark. Therefore, a correlation between those two scores should indicate the degree to which height is responsible for jump scores and thus how much (the remainder) is due to other factors (leg strength, timing, etc.)

In order to find the amount of correlation, we need a measure which will vary with that correlation. Multiplying the scores of each boy on the two factors will give us such a measure. If Tom is the tallest and touches the highest point, then his height multiplied by the height of his jump point will be the largest score possible for the group; and similarly if Dick is the shortest and reached the lowest point of anyone in the group, his height multiplied by that point will be the lowest score in the group.

If Joe, who is shorter, can touch the same jump height as Tom, we still would not get the maximum possible score when multiplying the two factors. Any deviation from the perfect relationship will lower the sum of these multiplications and give us a lesser degree of correlation.

There follow some examples of varying score possibilities.

As these examples are examined, it will be noted that deviation scores are used. Since we have two sets of scores, deviation scores are now indicated by the lower case letters x and y. Since scores on different tests have such varying ranges, we must compare how a person differs from the mean of a factor so that his score will be understandable to us. Although it may be obvious in these examples, in a larger group we would want to know if he were taller or shorter than the average of the group and whether or not his score was above average.

In example A, the correlation is perfect (the tallest boy has the highest score, etc.), the sum of the products of the deviation (Σ xy)

---

*In practice we attempt to eliminate this factor by subtracting reach height from jump height to obtain the jump-reach score.

EXAMPLE 26

	Height	Jump Height			
A	**X**	**Y**	**x**	**y**	**xy**
Tom	70	85	4	4	16
Joe	68	83	2	2	4
Sam	66	81	0	0	0
Bob	64	79	-2	-2	4
Dick	62	77	-4	-4	16
$(M_X = 66)$ $\Sigma X = 330$		$\Sigma Y = 405$ $(MY = 81)$			$\Sigma xy = 40$
B	**X**	**Y**			
Tom	70	77	4	-4	-16
Joe	68	79	2	-2	- 4
Sam	66	81	0	0	0
Bob	64	83	-2	2	- 4
Dick	62	85	-4	4	-16
					$\Sigma xy = -40$
C	**X**	**Y**			
Tom	70	81	4	0	0
Joe	68	77	2	-4	-8
Sam	66	85	0	4	0
Bob	64	79	-2	-2	4
Dick	62	83	-4	2	-8
					$\Sigma xy = -12$
D	**X**	**Y**			
Tom	70	83	4	2	8
Joe	68	85	2	4	8
Sam	66	81	0	0	0
Bob	64	77	-2	-4	8
Dick	62	79	-4	-2	8
					$\Sigma xy = 32$

is 40. In Example B the opposite relationships exist (the tallest boy has the lowest score, etc.), and Σ xy is -40.

Forty is the most Σ xy can be in this case and -40 is the least. Any score in between indicates a varying degree of relationship as in examples C and D. Note that the closer Σ xy approaches maximum (40) the greater is the relationship between height and jump score.

Since we might wish to compare the correlations of groups of different size (i.e., 20 people in one and 5 in another) it would seem wise to always divide Σ xy by N (in this case N = 5).

This number, $\dfrac{\Sigma\ xy}{N}$ would now seem to be a good indication of relationship. However, it is not a stable number because it varies with the tests and the units in which they are measured. Even these same scores translated to centimeters would give a different result than that gotten with scores in inches. The way to overcome this weakness is to divide the deviation scores by their standard deviations, e.g., $\frac{x}{SD_X}$ and $\frac{y}{SD_Y}$. This process will always provide similar scores (standard scores). For example, compare a test based on 100 with a mean of 50 and an SD of 10 with a test based on 10 with a mean of 5 and an SD of 1. A person receiving a score of 60 on the one and a score of 6 on the other would have deviation scores of 10 and 1. If we divide each by the standard deviation of the test we would have scores of $\frac{10}{10}$ = 1 and $\frac{1}{1}$ = 1. These scores are actually equivalent on these two tests—each being one SD to the right of the mean. When deviation scores are expressed in this way, scores on any test may be compared.

What we now have is a formula for correlation:

$$r = \frac{\Sigma\left(\frac{x}{SD_X} \times \frac{y}{SD_Y}\right)}{N} = \frac{\text{Sum of cross products of standard scores}}{N}$$

This formula is rather awkward however, and it may be reduced mathematically to:

$$r = \frac{\Sigma xy}{\sqrt{\Sigma x^2 \times \Sigma y^2}}$$

Now our original indication of relationship (Σxy) has been translated into a form always comparable, and always ranging between +1.00 and -1.00.

What we have done is to change each score into a standard score, multiply the two standard scores of each student, sum the results and divide by N, but we have by-passed many of these steps.

An r approaching +1.00, such as .90, indicates a high positive relationship between the tests or factors; actually it indicates that 81 percent (.90 squared) of the results on the one test are affected by the presence of the other factor although a causal relationship may not be assumed. A correlation of .20 although positive and showing some relationship actually only shows a possible 4 percent influence of one factor in the other.

Let us follow our example through and find the correlations for each. Note the columns needed to derive the sums needed.

EXAMPLE 27

A	X	Y	x	y	xy	x^2	y^2
Tom	70	85	4	4	16	16	16
Joe	68	83	2	2	4	4	4
Sam	66	81	0	0	0	0	0
Bob	64	79	-2	-2	4	4	4
Dick	62	77	-4	-4	16	16	16

$M_X = 66$ $\Sigma xy = 40$ $\Sigma x^2 = 40$ $\Sigma y^2 = 40$

$$r = \frac{\Sigma xy}{\sqrt{\Sigma x^2 \times \Sigma y^2}} = \frac{40}{\sqrt{40 \times 40}} = \frac{40}{40} = 1.00$$

B.	X	Y	x	y	xy	x^2	y^2
Tom	70	77	4	-4	-16	16	16
Joe	68	79	2	-2	-4	4	4
Sam	66	81	0	0	0	0	0
Bob	64	83	-2	2	-4	4	4
Dick	62	85	-4	4	-16	16	16

$\Sigma xy = -40$ $\Sigma x^2 = 40$ $\Sigma y^2 = 40$

$$r = \frac{\Sigma xy}{\sqrt{\Sigma x^2 \times \Sigma y^2}} = \frac{-40}{\sqrt{40 \times 40}} = \frac{-40}{40} = -1.00$$

C	X	Y	x	y	xy	x^2	y^2
Tom	70	81	4	0	0	16	0
Joe	68	77	2	-4	-8	4	16
Sam	66	85	0	4	0	0	16
Bob	64	79	-2	-2	4	4	4
Dick	62	83	-4	2	-8	16	4

$\Sigma xy = -12$ $\Sigma x^2 = 40$ $\Sigma y^2 = 40$

$$r = \frac{\Sigma xy}{\sqrt{\Sigma x^2 \times \Sigma y^2}} = \frac{-12}{\sqrt{40 \times 40}} = \frac{-12}{40} = -.30$$

D	X	Y	x	y	xy	x^2	y^2
Tom	70	83	4	2	8	16	4
Joe	68	85	2	4	8	4	16
Sam	66	81	0	0	0	0	0
Bob	64	77	-2	-4	8	4	16
Dick	62	79	-4	-2	8	16	4

$$\Sigma xy = 32 \quad \Sigma x^2 = 40 \quad \Sigma y^2 = 40$$

$$r = \frac{\Sigma xy}{\sqrt{\Sigma x^2 \times \Sigma y^2}} = \frac{32}{\sqrt{40 \times 40}} = \frac{32}{40} = .80$$

Parts A and B of example 27 are perfect correlations although Part B shows a perfect inverse relationship. Part C shows a low negative relationship (r = -.30) of only nine percent and we can only say that there is little or no relationship shown between height and jump height. Part D indicates a fairly high positive relationship (r = .80) of 64 percent.

Standard Error of the Difference Between Correlated Means

The formula which we have used for SE_D is actually a sub-formula from the general one for the standard error of any difference. In our particular case we were comparing scores of two different groups on the same test. However, we might wish to test on the basketball throw; follow that by a program of exercises designed to build arm and shoulder strength; and then test again to find out if the exercise influenced basketball throwing performance. The actual differences might not be as great as those existing between two different groups, but they would be as meaningful. For example if everyone improved even a little bit it would certainly indicate that the training program had been effective, and yet the difference between the means might be too small to pass the 5 percent level of confidence on our distribution of possible chance differences. Our present formula for SE_D might eliminate our obtained difference as not being great enough to be significant, therefore we must take into consideration the correlation between the first and second scores, and the formula now becomes:

$$SE_D = \sqrt{SE_{m_1}{}^2 + SE_{m_2}{}^2 - (2r_{12} SE_{m_1} SE_{m_2})}$$

EXAMPLE 28

Student	X	Y	x	y	xy	x^2	y^2
A	10	8	+4.5	+3	+13.5	20.25	9
B	9	10	+3.5	+5	+17.5	12.25	25
C	8	6	+2.5	+1	+ 2.5	6.25	1
D	7	3	+1.5	-2	- 3.0	2.25	4
E	6	8	+0.5	+3	+ 1.5	0.25	9
F	5	4	-0.5	-1	+ 0.5	0.25	1
G	4	4	-1.5	-1	+ 1.5	2.25	1
H	3	5	-2.5	0	0	6.25	0
I	2	1	-3.5	-4	+14.0	12.25	16
J	1	1	-4.5	-4	+18.0	20.25	16

$$\Sigma X = 55 \quad \Sigma Y = 50 \qquad \Sigma xy = 66.0 \quad \Sigma x^2 = 82.50 \quad \Sigma y^2 = 82$$

$$N = 10$$
$$M_x = 5.5$$
$$M_y = 5.0$$

$$r = \frac{\Sigma xy}{\sqrt{\Sigma x^2 \times \Sigma y^2}} = \frac{66}{\sqrt{82.50 \times 82}} = \frac{66}{\sqrt{6765}} =$$

$$\frac{66}{82.25} = .80$$

Note that we can find SD's and SE_m's from the figures now available.

When the correlation (r) is high it means that each student's score changed in a manner similar to that of each other student. For instance, each student increased his score, or for a perfect correlation each increased his score enough to remain in the same rank order as before.

If we look at the formula we will find that the higher "r" is the smaller will be the SE_D, because the number of which it is multiplying part ($2 \times r \times SE_{m_1} \times SE_{m_2}$) is subtracted from the number which was our previous SE_D $\sqrt{SE_{m_1}^2 + SE_{m_2}^2}$. This means that the SE_D of correlated scores will not be as large as with uncorrelated scores, and further, the higher the correlation the smaller it will be. When we now put it in the formula for $CR\left(\frac{D}{SE_D}\right)$ we find that the CR will be larger when SE_D is smaller, and in effect smaller differences

PROBLEM 10

Find the coefficient of correlation for the following scores:

Student	X	Y	x	y	xy	x^2	y^2
A	8	10					
B	5	6					
C	3	5					
D	2	1					
E	7	8					
F	6	5					
G	8	9					
H	7	8					
I	4	3					
j	10	10					
	$\Sigma X =$	$\Sigma Y =$			$\Sigma xy =$	$\Sigma x^2 =$	$\Sigma y^2 =$

$N =$

$M_x =$

$M_y =$

$r =$

between correlated scores can be as significant as larger differences on uncorrelated scores. It is important to use the proper formula when retesting the same group. Similarly it would be an error to use the SE_D formula for correlated means on scores which do *not* meet the criteria for correlated groups. Actually the formula

$$SE_D = \sqrt{SE_1{}^2 + SE_2{}^2 - 2r_{1\,2}\,SE_1\,SE_2}$$

is the general formula for comparing differences between any measures. In the case of two different groups, or the same group on different (uncorrelated) tests, r is zero (you need paired scores for a correlation) and therefore the entire last number would be zero leaving our original formula for uncorrelated scores.

If (in Example 29) we had not used the formula for correlated scores our SE_D would be .47 and $t = \dfrac{1.49}{.47} = 3.17$ which is less than half as large and might very well, in another problem, bring our difference into the area of sampling error.

EXAMPLE 29
OBSTACLE RACE

First Testing		Second Testing
M = 22.15		M = 20.66
SD = 2.24		SD = 2.38

$$N = 49$$
$$r = .80$$

$$SE_{mI} = \frac{2.24}{\sqrt{49}} = .32 \qquad\qquad SE_{mII} = \frac{2.38}{\sqrt{49}} = .34$$

$$SE_D = \sqrt{(.32)^2 + (.34)^2 - (2 \times .80 \times .32 \times .34)}$$

$$= \sqrt{.1024 + .1156 - (.174080)}$$

$$= \sqrt{.0439} = .21$$

$$D = 1.49$$

$$t = \frac{1.49}{.21} = 7.09 \qquad .01 \rangle p$$

EXAMPLE 30

M_1 = 50		M_2 = 56	
SE_{m1} = 2		SE_{m2} = 3	

$$r = .90$$

Using the formula for correlated scores:

$$SE_D = \sqrt{4 + 9 - (2 \times .90 \times 2 \times 3)} = \sqrt{2.2} = 1.48$$

$$t = \frac{6}{1.48} = 4.05$$

If we had used the formula for uncorrelated scores the CR would not have been significant.

$$(SE_D = 3.6; \quad t = 1.67).$$

PROBLEM 11

Find the SE_D for the following correlated scores:
Is the difference significant?_____

Student	X	Y	x	y	xy	x^2	y^2
A	8	10					
B	5	6					
C	3	5					
D	2	1					
E	7	8					
F	6	5					
G	7	9					
H	5	8					
I	4	3					
J	10	10					

$N =$ $\Sigma X =$ $\Sigma Y =$ $\Sigma xy =$ $\Sigma x^2 =$ $\Sigma y^2 =$

$M_x =$

$M_y =$ $D = M_x - M_y =$

$SD_x = \sqrt{\dfrac{\Sigma x^2}{N}} =$ $r = \dfrac{\Sigma xy}{\sqrt{\Sigma x^2 \times \Sigma y^2}} =$

$SD_y = \sqrt{\dfrac{\Sigma y^2}{N}} =$

$SE_{mx} = \dfrac{SD}{\sqrt{N}} =$ $SE_D = \sqrt{SE_{mx}^2 + SE_{my}^2 - (2 \times r \times SE_{mx} \times SE_{my})}$

$SE_{my} = \dfrac{SD}{\sqrt{N}} =$ $t = \dfrac{D}{SE_D}$

The Standard Error of the Difference Between Differences

If we can test before-and-after performance, as we could physical fitness, or skills with which our students have had some experience, we can measure improvement. Should we now wish to compare two methods of teaching or training, then we would wish to use one method with one group and the other method with a second group and test whether one group *improved* more than the other as a result of the method used. In such a case we need to test the significance of the difference between differences, administering the test to *each* group before and after training. With such a procedure, our difference between differences, (D_D) would be found by finding the differences between the pre and post means of each group, $(D_I = MI_{pre} - MI_{post})$ and $(D_{II} = MII_{pre} - MII_{post})$, and taking the D_D to be $D_I - D_{II}$.

The SE_{D_D} is found in the same manner as SE_D, using the SE_D's for each group in the formula:

$$SE_{D_D} = \sqrt{SE_{D_I}{}^2 + SE_{D_{II}}{}^2}$$

The critical ratio is then:

$$CR = \frac{D_D}{SE_{D_D}}$$

and our levels of confidence will be the same as we have used before.

The Experimental Design

We now have the statistical tools for an experimental design. Not only can we describe our scores and our group, but we can compare groups, or methods, or circumstances.

1. If we wished to establish the amount of relationship between two tests, or between a test and the quality being measured, we need only to find the correlation between the scores and interpret that correlation in terms of the percentage of relationship.

2. Perhaps we just want to know whether our group is improving as a result of the program. This can be determined through before-and-after testing, using the SE_D for correlated scores as the technique for determining the critical ratio.

3. Possibly we are interested in comparing our students with those at another school. For such a comparison we need to use the SE_D for uncorrelated scores in the critical ratio.

4. If we wished to try a new method of performing or teaching a skill, then we could divide our students into two groups, using the new method with one group and the old method with the other; compare the difference between the means of the two groups, allowing statistically for sampling error, and determine whether or not the new method was significantly superior to the old.

5. If the skill or ability is one which can be measured before as well as after training then the statistical technique is to use the standard error of the difference between differences to determine the effectiveness of the methods.

EXAMPLE 31

Group I		Group II	
$M_I = 40$	$M_{II} = 50$	$M_I = 45$	$M_{II} = 60$
pretest	posttest	pretest	posttest
$SE_{MI} = 2$	$SE_{MI} = 3$	$SE_{MII} = 2$	$SE_{MII} = 1.5$
pre	post	pre	post
	$r = .90$		$r = .80$

$$SE_{DII} = \sqrt{2^2 + 1.5^2 - 2 \times .80 \times 2 \times 1.5}$$

$$SE_{DI} = \sqrt{SE_{M_{pre}}^2 + SE_{M_{post}}^2 - 2r\, SE_{M_{pre}}\, SE_{M_{post}}}$$

$$= \sqrt{6.25 - 4.8}$$

$$= \sqrt{1.45}$$

$$= \sqrt{2^2 + 3^2 - 2 \times .90 \times 2 \times 3}$$

$$= 1.2$$

$$= \sqrt{13 - 10.8}$$

$$D = 15$$

$$= \sqrt{2.2}$$

$$= 1.5$$

$$D = M_{pre} - M_{post} = 10$$

Note that it is not necessary to the problem to find the SE_D's since the number under the square root in the SE_D *is* SE_D squared it may be put directly into the formula for SE_{D_D}.

$$SE_{D_D} = \sqrt{SE_{D_I}^2 + SE_{D_{II}}^2}$$

$$= \sqrt{1.5^2 + 1.2^2}$$

$$= \sqrt{2.25 + 1.44}$$

$$= \sqrt{3.69}$$

$$= 1.9$$

$$D_D = D_I - D_{II} = 5$$

$$CR = \frac{D_D}{SE_{D_D}} = \frac{5}{1.9} = 2.63$$

which is significant at the 1 percent level of confidence. Group II improved significantly over Group I.

Note that SE_D for correlated scores is used when measuring improvement of each group, but when comparing two groups there is no correlation and the formula for SE_D is that for uncorrelated scores.

PROBLEM 12

Find the significance of the difference between the differences for the following:

$M_I = 40$	$M_I = 50$	$M_{II} = 45$	$M_{II} = 60$
pre	post	pre	post
$SE_{MI} = 1$	$SE_{MI} = 1.5$	$SE_{MII} = 2$	$SE_{MII} = 1.2$
$r = .60$		$r = .90$	

CLUES IN EXPERIMENTAL DESIGN
CONTROL OF EXTRANEOUS VARIABLES

When designing an experiment it is necessary to eliminate or control as many extraneous variables as possible since factors not associated with the experiment can affect the performance of the groups.

If the experiment can be completed in one day it is possible to eliminate problems associated with changes in the health status of subjects, absences, and changes in testing conditions (weather, etc.). There are cases however when, even with sufficient time, it would be unwise to administer both parts of an experiment on the same day. An example of such a time would be when testing strength or endurance was part of the design, and the students were expected to give maximum effort. In such a case, fatigue would become a new variable influencing performance on subsequent tasks. Of course, when the problem involves improvement, the second testing is given after the training program and necessarily requires a later date. It is important, however, to try to duplicate conditions on all testing.

The effect of performing one task on the performance of a second task must be taken into consideration. To balance this effect, the group can be divided and the order of the tests alternated, giving Test A first and Test B second to one half of the group, and Test B first with Test A second, to the other half of the group.

THE EFFECT OF MOTIVATING CONDITIONS

Motivation is another factor to be considered in any testing situation. If a student is not trying to perform as well as possible, his score will not reflect his ability. Securing the interest and cooperation of the group is vital. Of course, if we are testing the effect of different motivational conditions, then they are the experimental variables; otherwise, the atmosphere of the testing situation is an extraneous variable which needs to be controlled.

CONSISTENCY OF TESTING PROCEDURES

Although it is not always practical, it is appropriate, when possible, to have the same person administer any one test to all subjects. This is not so necessary if the objectivity of the test is very high, but consistency in instructions and scoring is essential.

EXAMPLE 32

Comparison of Right or Left Preference with Running Skill Involving Turning Right or Left

Equipment Needed: 1 Stop watch

Procedure

Race course as diagrammed

1. Half of group run to right first and to left second.
2. Other half run to left first and to right second.
3. List scores according to hand preference.

    X = Preferred hand
    Y = Non-preferred hand

Problem

Measure the difference between scores (Difference between correlated means).

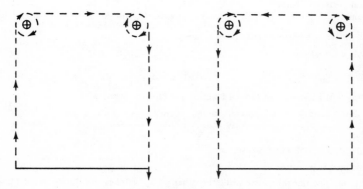

Figure 5.9

EXAMPLE 33

Effect of Competition on Performance

Equipment needed: 2 stop watches, straight race course, and reasonable distance.

Procedure

Run races twice (pair on basis of previous scores)

1. Half of group run alone first, then with competition.

2. Other half run with competition first, then alone.

Problem

Measure difference between methods

X = Alone

Y = With Competition

Difference between correlated means.

EXAMPLE 34

Comparison of Grip Strength With Performance of a Skill

Equipment Needed: Hand dynamometer, stop watches, basketballs.

Procedure

1. Measure right and left grip strength with the hand dynamometer.

2. Test-Bounce ball two 30-second periods (total score).

3. Half of group do preferred hand first and non-preferred second. Other half do non-preferred hand first and preferred second.

Problem

1. Compare strength of preferred with non-preferred hand.

2. Compare skill of preferred with non-preferred hand.

3. Compare strength with skill.

    a. Preferred hand.
    b. Non-preferred hand.
    c. Combine all scores (strength = total right and left, and skill = total right and left).

1 and 2—difference between correlated means

3—Simple correlations

EXAMPLE 35

Comparison of Efficiency of Mental Practice and Physical Practice

Equipment needed: Obstacle course, own design, stop watches.

Procedure

1. Total group run obstacle course.

2. Divide into two groups.

3. One group practice on course while the other group watches and thinks (mental practice).

4. Total group run course again.

Problem

Compare improvements of the two groups. Difference between differences.

chapter

6

Test Construction

Skill Test Construction

There is no reason why the instructor cannot construct his own skill tests; he need only follow these steps:

1. Determine the component skills in the activity.
   Example: Basketball might include shooting, passing, and dribbling.

2. Devise tests of those skills.
   Example: *Shooting*: Any number of possibilities exist, such as one-handed push shots from ten marked positions. Scored according to number of successes. *Passing:* Wall-pass in which student throws ball against wall from behind restraining line. Scored

239

according to number of hits in 30 seconds.* *Dribbling:* Set up an obstacle course; students dribble through course. Scored according to time needed to complete the course.

3. Administer tests to a large group.

4. Validate tests by comparing scores on each test with a criterion. Validity may be determined in the following ways:

   a. In an individual sport such as tennis singles, validity may be determined by correlating test scores with games won in a round robin tournament.

   b. Have students evaluated on their play by expert judges. An expert judge would be the physical education instructor, other physical education teachers, and coaches. If necessary, the judgment of the instructor would be sufficient; however, it would be better to have additional judges and combine their scores. Judges may score players on any one of several systems. Normally the judges should have a range of choices (1 to 7, or A+ to D-), in order to make sufficient differentiation possible (see construction of rating scales and the 12-point system of grades). Judges' scores and test scores are correlated in order to determine validity.

5. Evaluate validities and combine tests since no one skill represents the entire ability. Validities will not necessarily be high; however, when all tests are combined the single battery might well provide a good validity. In order to combine the tests without more extensive statistical procedures, scores must be converted to the same scale; standard scores, T-scores for example. We may now add together a student's standard scores and thus determine for him a battery score.

6. Validate battery. The battery score may now be used with the ratings to find the validity of the battery.

7. Weighting items. Through item analysis and multiple correlation techniques, the best weights for each of the tests in the battery can be found; however, the instructor might wish to count one test more than another in the battery score.

   Example: Shooting 3, dribbling 2, and passing 1. The instructor can use his judgment in making these weights or he might use the percentage of relationship indicated by the validities of the sepa-

---

*Skill tests should not involve another person, since you are then measuring the weaker person.

rate tests. For example, if the validities were: shooting .60, passing .30, and dribbling .40, these indicate percentages of:

Shooting $r = .60—36\%$ Weight = 4
Passing $r = .30— 9\%$ Weight = 1
Dribbling $r = .40—16\%$ Weight = 2

Rounding the percentages would provide weights of 4, 1, and 2. A student's standard score could then be multiplied by the weight, and his battery score would be the total of the weighted test scores. A new correlation should then be found to determine whether or not the weights improved the validity. Test validities of .60, .40, and .30 might well provide a battery validity of .70 or higher. We need to know this validity to determine the weight which the skill test battery will carry in the grade. A validity of .70 still represents only a 49 percent relationship and so should not comprise the whole grade.

Construction of Written Tests

Rate the last written test which you took. Did it examine knowledge and understanding of the subject or was it superficial? Were the instructions clear or was it necessary to ask what was expected? Were the questions fair or tricky? Was the emphasis of the test about equivalent to that given during instruction? Was there variety in the types of questions? If all of these questions can be answered positively it was a good test and we would do well to use it as an example.

Most written tests in physical education are, of necessity, teacher-made. There are very few standardized knowledge tests in physical education, and since the instructor will be testing his students on what he taught them it is only proper that the test be written *for them* and reflect his teaching emphasis.

CONSTRUCTION OF WRITTEN TEST QUESTIONS

The first step in writing a test is to understand how to construct different types of questions, their advantages and disadvantages and their uses in measuring knowledge and understanding.

ALTERNATE RESPONSE

This type of question usually requires the student to judge whether the statement is true or false, although any format which provides only two choices fits in this category, e.g., fair or foul, point or side out. The advantage of alternate-response questions is that a great amount of material may be covered in a relatively short test-taking time. Questions can be written rather quickly but there are hazards. A good true-false question is sometimes hard to construct because:

1. The instructor must avoid including leading words such as seldom, always, usually, and never. These terms betray the proper response.

   Examples:

   A. There are only two types of serves in volleyball.

   B. The "frog kick" is always used with the breast stroke.

   Merely by guessing it would be logical to rate each of these questions false because of the cue words "only" and "always."

2. The question should involve only one idea.

   Examples:

   A. A ball touching the top of the net and falling fair is in play, unless it is a serve.

   B. A foul ball is considered to be a strike except if it is the third strike, or if it is caught.

   This information could be better gained through two or more questions or with a different type of question.

3. A question should not be partly true and partly false.

   Examples:

   A. The server (in tennis) must stand between the center mark and the sideline.

   B. The baserunner is out if he is hit by a batted ball.

   Neither of these are good questions since not enough information is given; and since giving more information would involve additional concepts it would be better to use a different type question for this information.

4. Questions should be stated in positive terms. If a negative is necessary it should be underlined. Watch out for double negatives.

   Examples:

   A. If the pitcher "balks" baserunners are not allowed to advance one base.

   B. A baserunner does not have to be tagged if he is not forced.

   Both of these questions would be better stated if the negatives were omitted entirely.

5. Alternate-response questions do *not* lend themselves well to questions of opinion.

Examples:

A. The interlocking grip is preferable to the overlapping grip.

B. It is better to have played and lost than never to have played at all.

Of course students will probably be able to answer according to what they think the instructor believes, but should they happen to believe otherwise and answer that way, can their answer be marked wrong?

6. Avoid such general terms as several, many, some. Questions should be specific regarding amounts or numbers.

Examples:

A. There are several ways to score in soccer.

B. Some fouls are considered to be team fouls.

These are better written with a number such as "two ways to score," or a specific such as "substitution fouls are considered."

EXAMPLE 36
ALTERNATE RESPONSE

Directions: True-False. Circle the letter T if the statement is true, circle the letter F if the statement is false.

SWIMMING

T F 1. The overarm stroke is an example of the use of opposite force in producing momentum.

T F 2. In the underwater breast stroke the arms and legs power alternately.

ELEMENTARY BACKSTROKE

T F 1. Kick is similar to that of the crawl stroke.

T F 2. Breath control is difficult to learn in this stroke.

T F 3. Requires a minimum amount of energy.

T F 4. Arms recover out of the water.

T F 5. Legs and arms recover simultaneously.

MATCHING

Matching questions are most useful for identification of people, places, definitions, and rules. This type of question presents two or three lists of items and the student is asked to match items on the second and/or third lists with items on the first list. There are three good formats for matching questions:

1. **Imperfect.** In this format more items are provided in the second list than are in the first list. This helps reduce guessing, one of the disadvantages of matching questions. The number of items in a list should be limited to no more than 15 and no fewer than 5, and items in any one question should be homogeneous in topic. For example: if you wished to ask questions about people and places, it would be better to use two questions, one for each topic, rather than combine both into one question.

EXAMPLE 37

Directions: Place the *letter* of the appropriate organization in the space provided.

_____ 1. Organization governing amateur sports in America.

_____ 2. Organization governing college athletics in America.

_____ 3. National professional physical education association.

_____ 4. Governs women's collegiate athletics.

_____ 5. Rules governing body for golf.

(a) AAHPER
(b) AAU
(c) DGWS
(d) NCAA
(e) USGA
(f) USLTA

Directions: Place the *letter* of the appropriate person in the space provided to the left of each statement.

_____ 1. Grandfather of physical education.

_____ 2. First president of P.E. professional organization.

_____ 3. Thought aim of education was happiness.

_____ 4. Instrumental in growth of measurement in physical education.

_____ 5. Developed athletic achievement tests with YMCA.

_____ 6. Founded interpretive dancing.

_____ 7. Gave first "modern dance" concert.

_____ 8. Day's order of exercises in public schools.

(a) Aristotle
(b) Catherine Beecher
(c) Isadora Duncan
(d) Martha Graham
(e) Luther Gulick
(f) Guts Muth
(g) Margaret H'Doubler
(h) Edward Hitchcock
(i) Dio Lewis
(j) Dudley Sargent
(k) Jesse F. Williams

It is also helpful to alphabetize items on the second list or to put them in some logical order.

2. Classification. This format provides a limited number of items on the second list, but may provide any number of items on list one, with items from the second list used more than once. This type of question is excellent for situations involving the application of rules.

EXAMPLE 38
CLASSIFICATION
VOLLEYBALL

Directions: Indicate the official's decision in the following situations, using the key letters for your answers. There is only one best answer. Assume that no conditions exist other than those stated.

     P—point   L—Legal, or play continues

     SO—side out   R—re-serve, or serve over

_____ 1. Server steps on the end line as the ball leaves her fist.

_____ 2. On the service, the ball touches the top of the net and lands on the boundary line of the receiving team's court.

_____ 3. A player on the receiving team spikes the ball before it crosses to her side of the net. She does not touch the net.

_____ 4. A forward on the serving team, in spiking the ball, returns to the floor across the center line. On the same play, a forward of the receiving team who attempts to block the ball steps on the center line.

_____ 5. As a player on the serving team attempts to contact the ball, it touches her upper arm.

SOCCER

Directions: Place the appropriate letter in the space provided.

     A—Free kick for opposing team   E—Free kick on penalty circle

     B—Kick-in for opposing team   F—Penalty kick

     C—Roll in   G—No penalty

     D—Corner kick   H—Score

_____ 1. On a kick-in player A dribbles the ball rather than kicking it.

_____ 2. A team "B" player, taking a kick in, sends the ball between the goal posts.

_____ 3. "A" is tackling "B" who has the ball, it goes out of bounds off both players.

_____ 4. During play the ball is lofted into the air, and the left inner bounces it off his knee through the goal posts.

Note that it is helpful to provide an item indicating that the play is fair, or not an infraction of the rules.

3. Multiple lists. This format provides more than one list, each of which is to be matched with the items in list one. You might wish to use this type to match people, places, and events; or, using the classification format, to determine the effect of the situation on two groups, or to identify decision and result.

EXAMPLE 39

SOFTBALL

Directions: Each statement describes a situation in which the batter and baserunners may be involved. Find the number which gives the correct ruling for the batter and the baserunner from the code "Batter" and "Baserunner" and place that number in the parenthesis provided on the answer sheet.

Example: There is one out and a runner on first base. Batter hits the ball between home and first. The ball rolls into foul territory and stops.

        (2) Batter   (6) Baserunner

CODE

**BATTER OR
BATTER-BASERUNNER**

(1) Is out

(2) Strike is called

(3) Ball is called

(4) Becomes baserunner with liability of being put out.

(5) Becomes baserunner for one base without liability of being put out.

(6) Entitled to 2 or more bases without liability of being put out.

(7) Does not affect.

BASERUNNER

(1) Is out

(2) May advance any number of bases with liability of being put out.

(3) Advance limited to one base with liability of being put out.

(4) Entitled to one base without liability of being put out.

(5) Entitled to two or more bases without liability of being put out.

(6) Must return to base, or to last legally held base.

1. The pitcher makes a motion to pitch without immediately delivering the ball to the batter. Runner is on second.

2. The batter is struck by a pitched ball which he tried to avoid. The runner on second goes to third base.

3. A runner is on second. The batter hits a ball which lands outside third base line but rolls into the infield just as it reaches third base.

4. The batter with two strikes swings but misses a fairly delivered pitch, and the catcher misses the ball. There is one out and a runner on second.

SHORT ANSWER AND COMPLETION

Short answer and completion questions can be similar to matching questions, except that the first or second list is not given. This makes the questions more difficult since recall is necessary.

EXAMPLE 40

SOCCER

Directions: Write the official's decision and result in the space provided to the left of each statement.

_____ 1. On a kick-in player A dribbles the ball rather than kicking it.

_____ 2. The attacking team sends the ball over the end line not between the goal posts.

_____ 3. "A" is tackling "B" who has the ball, it goes out of bounds off both players.

This type question is also good to question information requiring multiple responses.

EXAMPLE 41

The three fencing weapons are:

1. _____   3. _____

2. _____

Another use of completion questions is for scoring.

EXAMPLE 42
TENNIS

Directions: Give the score at the end of the indicated points.
         A is serving.

Point.......	(1)	(2)	(3)	(4)	(5)	(6)	(7)	(8)	(9)
_____	A	A	B	A					
_____	B	A	A	B	B	A	A		
_____	A	A							
_____	B	B	A	A	B				
_____	B								
_____	A	A	B	B	B	A	A	A	

These questions can be set up as a progression; however, it is important to note that one error will affect subsequent answers, and the teacher must make the appropriate adjustment to all subsequent answers when grading.

EXAMPLE 43

Directions: Give the score of the following game as each point is played.

Point......	(1)	(2)	(3)	(4)	(6)	(7)	(8)
_____	A						
_____		B					
_____			A				
_____				B			

Note: It is poor practice to excerpt a statement from the rule book, leaving a word blank; this encourages rote learning and sometimes is

confusing to the point of comedy, as: The first rule in tennis is to
_____ the _____ in the _____.

MULTIPLE CHOICE

This is the most highly regarded type of question because it can
measure applications of information as opposed to memorization; it
may require reasoning through more than one step, and, although
alternatives are given, it is not easy to guess the best answer. This
applies when the question is well constructed, but herein lies the
catch, for good multiple choice questions are the most difficult to
construct because while there should be at least three and preferably
four alternatives and all alternatives must reasonably apply there is
nevertheless only one *best* answer. If the answer is obvious, it would
be better to ask the question in some other form.

Some hints on construction of multiple choice questions:

1. State the problem as simply as possible, preferably in positive
   terms. If a negative is necessary, *underline the negative.*

2. Be careful not to repeat phrasing from the question in an alternative.

3. Alternatives should be approximately the same length in the same
   tense and person.

EXAMPLE 44
SOFTBALL

Directions: Place the letter of the appropriate response in the space provided to the left of
the questions. There is only *one* best answer.

With the score tied, bases loaded and no outs, the ball is hit to short stop. He should
_____ throw to:

a. home

b. first base

c. the nearest base

d. second, in order to make a double play.

SWIMMING

_____ To recover to the standing position from a back float you should:

a. push head forward, pull knees to chest, scoop hands down and back, then up.

b. push head back, pull knees to chest, scoop hands down and back, then up.

c. push head forward, extend knees and arch back, scoop hands up and then down
and back.

d. push head backward, pull knees to chest, scoop hands up and then down and back.

4. Usually the use of "all of these" or "none of the above" does *not* present a reasonable alternative, or gives itself away as the best alternative.

SPECIAL FORMATS: DIAGRAMS, DRAWINGS, ETC.

Some information is best examined through the use of such special formats as diagrams and drawings. These include court lines, player positions, and tournament brackets.

Special formats may be set up as matching or multiple choice questions for ease of scoring. It is unwise to have the student draw in any or all of the material since it may become necessary to decide whether he just doesn't know the answer or he can't draw, and many can't.

EXAMPLE 45
TENNIS

Match the flight of the ball with the stroke. Place the letter of the appropriate flight in the space provided to the left of the stroke.

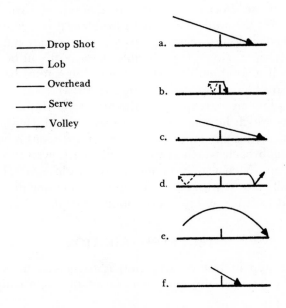

_____ Drop Shot

_____ Lob

_____ Overhead

_____ Serve

_____ Volley

ESSAY

This type of question has many disadvantages; however, when used by an experienced teacher, an essay question can shed light on the student's grasp of the problem and his depth of understanding.

EXAMPLE 46
POSTURAL DEVIATIONS

Directions: Identify each deviation in the space provided.

1. _____

2. _____

3. _____

4. _____

5. _____

If we are merely seeking to know if the student has acquired the facts, we can use short answer or objective type questions; however, should we wish the student to solve a problem through application of facts and recognition of relationships, our choices are multiple choice or essay. Multiple choice is preferable because it can be more easily scored, but if a good multiple choice question cannot be constructed around the problem, then essay is the answer.

When grading an essay question the instructor should have in mind some points which he might expect to be covered. He should beware however, of setting his mind too much for a student might well take a different approach which is worthy of merit, even though it might not be the approach which the instructor would have taken. Grading is most easily accomplished by noting the number of points made, giving credit for each and perhaps double or triple credit for some.

TEST CONSTRUCTION

The first step in test construction is to determine just what we want to test. This usually falls into one of the following categories:

1. Rules and their applications

2. Techniques

3. Courts, equipment, history, background, and definitions

4. Strategies

5. Scoring

We next consider the types of questions best suited to measure each. Although almost all types of questions can be written for each category, the following have been very successful:

1. Rules and their application—classification
2. Scoring—completion
3. Courts, equipment—special format
4. History and definitions—matching
5. Techniques—alternate response
6. Strategy—multiple-choice, matching, essay

The third step is to write the questions, being careful that one question doesn't contain a clue to the answer to another question, and attempting to have variety in the types of questions.

We must now decide the percent or weight each category should have in the test. This is determined by the amount of emphasis given in our teaching, and whether or not the written test will be the only time a category is measured. We will be grading, at other times, the student's performance of techniques and to some extent his strategy and application of rules in the game situation; whereas there may be no other opportunity to measure his knowledge of the background and history of the sport, selection and use of equipment, and possibly, scoring. Of course, history and equipment probably receive a minor degree of emphasis in our teaching, and certainly we would want to further probe our students' understanding of techniques, rules, and strategies, which are major parts of our teaching.

Weights might well vary from one sport to another since, for example, rules and strategies are more complicated in softball than in tennis, while swimming is primarily technique with considerable emphasis on safety and physical principles related to movement in the water.

Weightings may be accomplished by limiting the number of questions relating to each category, or giving different values to questions on each category with the percentage of the total score reflecting the emphasis.

The instructor should also consider the difficulty level of each type of question. The types may be ranked approximately as follows according to difficulty and opportunity to guess correctly.

1. Alternate Response   Easiest
2. Matching and Special Format
3. Completion Classification and Multiple Choice
4. Essay   Most Difficult

Note that unless the examiner is skilled at grading essay questions he may be taken in by a student who can pad his answer sufficiently to leave the impression that he knows more than he does.

Questions might be weighted by the numerical values given in the above ranking.

We may now either use different types of questions for each category, writing enough questions for each to provide the proper emphasis, or after having written questions of all types check the total points given to each category and if necessary adjust our questions to conform with our emphasis.

EXAMPLE 47

Desired Percentage	Category	Type Questions	Weight	Number Questions	Total Points
20	Rules	Classification	3	7	21
15	Scoring	Completion	3	5	15
15	Termin- ology, History & Background	Matching	2	7	14
20	Techniques	Alternate- Response	1	20	20
30	Strategy	Multiple- Choice	3	10	30
					100

It is not at all necessary for a test to add up to 100 points. In a major examination more questions should be included adding some variety to the types of questions used in some of the categories as in the following example.

The ratios of points to desired percentages remain approximately equivalent.

One should also consider that often we give more than one test, so no one test need contain all of the categories to be finally evaluated.

FURTHER HINTS ON TEST CONSTRUCTION

1. Instructions should be clear, stating specifically how the question is to be answered.

EXAMPLE 48

Desired Percentage	Category	Type Questions	Weight	Number Questions	Total Points
20	Rules	Classification	3	15	45
15	Scoring	Completion	3	5	15
		Special Format	7 items 1 pt. each	1	7
15	Terminology, History	Completion	3	5	15
		Matching	2	10	20
20	Techniques	Alternate-Response	1	30	30
		Special Format	2	5	10
30	Strategy	Multiple-Choice	3	10	30
		Matching	2	10	20
		Essay	4	2	8
					200

2. There should be about an equal number of right and wrong alternate-response questions and they should be in no particular order.

3. When preparing short answer questions all possible answers should be listed, such as alternate terms, and the instructor should be prepared to accept one of which he had not thought.

4. Any one essay question should be graded for all papers at one sitting if at all possible.

Test Analysis

A test should provide a fairly normal distribution of grades. Of course we will not always find the mean at the mid-point. It is very difficult to design a perfect test, but if the group is distributed in such a way as to find a few students at the extremes with the majority of scores around the mean then we have a discriminating test.

Test questions will vary in their ability to discriminate, and a good test will contain questions which range in this ability in a proportion similar to the normal distribution. There should be a few questions which only the better students will be able to answer and a few questions which almost all students will answer; the majority of questions should fall in the middle area of discrimination. A non-discriminatory question is one which:

1. Almost all students answer correctly.

2. Virtually none of the students can answer, or

3. Is answered correctly by the poorer students and missed by the better students.

The latter result would indicate that either the key was mismarked, or that a misleading statement existed in the question which caused the perceptive student to choose another answer. Poor questions should either be thrown out or rewritten.

In order to determine how well questions discriminate we use the process of item analysis. Should we be writing a test for purposes of publication the Flanagan (3) method of item analysis is recommended, however, a simpler method reported by Scott & French (7) will be presented here. This method is quite sufficient for use with teacher-made tests; however it should be used only if there are a large number (approximately 100) of answer sheets. The steps are as follows:

1. Select the top 29 percent of answer sheets, based on total test scores.

2. Select the bottom 29 percent on the same basis.

3. Prepare a tally sheet on which are indicated the number of correct responses for each group on each question, as in Figure 6.1.

N Upper = _____   N Lower = _____

Question	1		2	3	4	5	6
	ID		ID	ID	ID	ID	ID
	DR		DR	DR	DR	DR	DR
	7		8	9	10	11	12
	ID		ID	ID	ID	ID	ID
	DR		DR	DR	DR	DR	DR

Figure 6.1.

Supply columns in which to record Index of Discrimination (ID), and Difficulty Rating (DR) for each question.

4. Index of Discrimination—

$$ID = \frac{\text{number right in Upper group} - \text{number right in Lower group}}{\text{Number in one group}}$$

EXAMPLE 49

With N Upper and N Lower equalling 29*

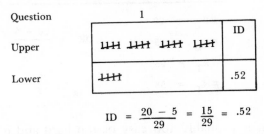

Question	1	
		ID
Upper	⫫⫫ ⫫⫫ ⫫⫫ ⫫⫫	
Lower	⫫⫫	.52

$$ID = \frac{20 - 5}{29} = \frac{15}{29} = .52$$

* (N for each group should be the same, if there were 100 papers N would equal 29 (29% of 100).

This figure is similar to a validity coefficient in that it indicates how valid the item is in relation to the entire test. The maximum ID would be +1.00, where all of the upper group answered the questions correctly and none of the lower group did so. A negative ID would indicate that the question did just what we did not want it to do (more lower group answered correctly than in the upper group), and such a question detracts from the validity of the entire test. An ID over +.20 is acceptable; below +.15 is not acceptable, and the question should be rewritten or thrown out. ID's between +.15 and +.19 are questionable.

5. Difficulty Rating—

$$DR = \frac{\text{Number right in Upper group} + \text{number right in Lower Group}}{\text{N Both Groups}}$$

$$= \frac{\text{Number } R_T}{N_T}$$

The higher the percentage of the total group answering the question correctly, the easier is the question. We would wish our test to contain a range, and a few difficult questions; however, a DR of more than 90 percent or less than 10 percent would indicate that

In our example:

EXAMPLE 50

Question . . . . .

		ID	DR
Upper	~~1111~~ ~~1111~~ ~~1111~~ ~~1111~~		
		.52	43%
Lower	~~1111~~		

$$\#R_U = 20$$
$$\#R_L = 5 \qquad DR = \frac{20 + 5}{58}$$
$$\#R_T = 25$$
$$\#N_T = 58 \qquad = \frac{25}{58} = 43\%$$

the question is probably too easy or too hard and is therefore a question of doubtful value.

6. Study the results to determine necessary revisions. Questions with poor ID's and/or DR's should be thrown out or rewritten. If there are more questions than necessary, a better test can be formed by eliminating the poor items entirely; however, in order to include sufficient questions for our categories of instruction, we may have to rewrite or write new questions to replace those eliminated. If the scores of the group did not approximate a normal distribution, we may adjust our test by making our new test according to the difficulty ratings with approximately the following percentages of the remaining good questions falling in each difficulty range.

TABLE 6.1

% of Questions		DR		
4	10	81	—	90
24	20	66	—	80
44 or	40	36	—	65
24	20	21	—	35
4	10	10	—	20

This will probably necessitate the elimination of some good questions, usually in the direction of the mean. If the mean was too high, thereby limiting a good distribution at the upper end of the scale, the test was too easy and we would eliminate some of the easier questions (high DR's). The choice then should hinge on the ID's of the items in question, keeping those with higher indices of discrimination.

EXAMPLE 51

Question		1	ID	DR
Upper		卌 卌 卌 卌	.52	43%
Lower		卌		

Question		8	ID	DR
Upper		卌 卌 卌 11	.31	43%
Lower		卌 111		

In this example both items possess DR's of 43 percent but question 1 has a higher index of discrimination and would be preferable.

PROBLEM 13

Find the index of discrimination and the difficulty rating for each of the following questions.

N Upper = 30   N Lower = 30

Question	1		2		3	
Upper	25	ID	30	ID	5	ID
Lower	10	DR	5	DR	15	DR

	4		5		6	
Upper	4	ID	15	ID	28	ID
Lower	1	DR	15	DR	20	DR

ANALYSIS OF MULTIPLE–CHOICE QUESTIONS

It was noted earlier that all alternatives in a multiple-choice question should be reasonable choices; therefore, if an alternative is not chosen by anyone it is serving no purpose and should be re-written. Multiple-choice questions may be analyzed at the same time we are analyzing our test by tallying the number of times each alternative was chosen by each group.

EXAMPLE 52

Question 10

	A	B	C	D	E	
Upper	111	1111	卌 卌 卌	卌 11		ID = .34
Lower	卌 1	卌 1	卌	卌 卌	11	DR = 34%

*C is correct answer

Question 11

	A	B	C	D	E	
Upper	卌 卌 卌 卌	111	11	1111		ID = .34
Lower	卌 卌	卌 11	卌 11	卌		DR = 52%

*A is correct answer

In this example question 10 is a good question; item E is the weakest, but at least 2 percent of the students chose it, which is considered sufficient. Question 11, however, contains a non-functioning item; since no one chose item E, it should either be eliminated or re-written. These questions have the following indices of discrimination and difficulty ratings:

$$\text{Question 10:} \quad \text{ID} = .34$$
$$\text{DR} = 34\%$$
$$\text{Question 11:} \quad \text{ID} = .34$$
$$\text{DR} = 52\%$$

It is interesting to note that the difference is in difficulty, which might be attributed to the non-functioning item. Question 11 is easier because it really only has four functioning alternatives while question 10 offers five choices. In a case where there are only three alternatives, and one is not functioning, we might do well to re-write the question in another format such as alternate response.

Scoring and Answer Sheets

There are three good ways to provide answer spaces for your tests, and each has advantages and disadvantages.

1. Answers on the test itself. Providing answer blanks on the test is advantageous to the student since the question and answer are in the same place; and he is not likely to place his answer in the wrong place. It is also helpful when the student is reviewing the test later to have both question and answer together. The disadvantages to this method are:
   a. The test is not reusable.
   b. It is more difficult to grade than an answer sheet. When spaces are provided on the test they should be placed along the margin opposite the question for ease of grading. Completions may be indicated in the body of the question with the number of the question.

EXAMPLE 53
FENCING

_____ 26. Right of way is established by (26) or (27).

_____ 27.

_____ 28. A reposte should be made immediately after you

  (28) an attack.

2. Answer sheets providing spaces in which the student writes the answer. This type allows the test to be used again and is easier to grade since it eliminates page turning.

3. Separate answer sheets containing all choices with the student's choice to be circled, crossed out, or filled in. This type permits use of an overlay scoring key with the correct response cut out and a mark made when the right answer is not indicated. This method of scoring is the quickest of the three but does not allow for

EXAMPLE 54

ANSWER SHEET

Class _____   Name _____

1. _____   26. _____

2. _____   27. _____

3. _____   28. _____

4. _____   29. _____

5. _____   30. _____

6. _____   31. _____

completion and short answer questions. This type answer sheet is very good when item analysis is planned.

EXAMPLE 55

ANSWER SHEET

4. Combinations of two and three are possible when the answer sheet is designed to fit the test.

EXAMPLE 56
SOFTBALL ANSWER SHEET

Class _____   Name _____

1.   ( )   Batter
      ( )   Baserunner
      ( )   Ball in play
      ( )   Ball is dead

2.   ( )   Batter
      ( )   Baserunner
      ( )   Ball in play
      ( )   Ball is dead

3.   ( )   Batter
      ( )   Baserunner
      ( )   Ball in play
      ( )   Ball is deal

11.   ( )   Batter
      ( )   Baserunner
      ( )   Ball in play
      ( )   Ball is dead

12.   ( )   Batter
      ( )   Baserunner
      ( )   Ball in play
      ( )   Ball is dead

13.   ( )   Batter
      ( )   Baserunner
      ( )   Ball in play
      ( )   Ball is deal

1._____ 21._____

2._____ 22._____

3._____ 23._____

4._____ 24._____

5._____ 25._____

6._____ 26._____

7._____ 27._____

	T a	F b	c	d	e				
1.	☐	☐	☐	☐	☐	33.		67.	
2.	☐	☐	☐	☐	☐	34.		68.	
3.	☐	☐	☐	☐	☐	35.		69.	
4.	☐	☐	☐	☐	☐	36.		70.	
5.	☐	☐	☐	☐	☐	37.		71.	
6.	☐	☐	☐	☐	☐	38.		72.	
7.	☐	☐	☐	☐	☐	39.		73.	
8.	☐	☐	☐	☐	☐	40. __ __ __ __ __		74. __ __ __ __ __	

chapter

7

Grading

Any teacher may be criticized for his or her grading practices and this is increasingly true as the pressure for grades continues to mount. So much depends today on a student's scholastic record. Secondary school is no longer a place for growing up and absorbing the cultural heritage—it's the testing ground which determines the direction of one's academic and vocational future. Students have a legitimate concern with methods of assigning grades.

Physical education grades have always been suspect. Some persons from other disciplines believe we tend to grade too leniently, others are critical because *"A"* students may not make *"A's"* in physical education. Some students don't understand or believe in the basis for the grade, and so naturally resent a poor grade and its effect on their point hour ratio.

We are not different from the other disciplines in the necessity to justify our grades. In some objectivity is fully expected—either you understand and can solve the math problem or you can't. It may be argued that in a like manner either you understand and can perform a skill or you can't. We feel, however, that there is more to be gained from learning a skill than knowledge and muscular control, because we still believe in the growth process occurring in any education endeavor: We believe in and try to promote social, emotional, and personal development in our students. In spite of the pressure for vocational preparation in school we know that school is a place where the major event, the dominating occurrence, perhaps the only real reason for being, is the student's search for identity, a place for growing up. As long as we believe this, and we teach for it, then we are faced with the necessity of assigning grades with reference to the accomplishment of all of the things we are teaching.

Perhaps we do not need to assign grades which reflect personal and social development; perhaps it is enough to encourage and promote these things and limit our grades to the degree of mastery of the more specific materials with which we work. We are faced with a dilemma, an almost unsurmountable dilemma, for our major problem lies in the variety of factors to be measured and in the difficulty of measuring some of those factors. In any event, we must know what we are trying to accomplish and be able to assess how well those objectives are being met—so let us get down to practicalities.

Any grade should reflect our objectives; how much of the grade is based on any one factor is a result of our philosophy and our belief in that factor's importance. The grade should indicate what we are measuring, our evaluation instruments should be valid, and we should be able to interpret the grade and make it understandable.

Measurable Factors

The factors which lend themselves to measurement can be divided into three categories:

1. Physical:
   a. Skill
   b. Fitness
   c. Motor Ability
   d. Game Performance
   e. Posture

2. Mental: Knowledge and Understanding of:

   a. Rules
   b. Performance
   c. Movement
   d. Strategy
   e. History
   f. Techniques
   g. Fitness
   h. Place of Physical Education in the School Program
   i. Conditioning
   j. Health and Safety

3. Social:

   a. Attitude
   b. Appreciation
   c. Sportsmanship
   d. Cooperation
   e. Citizenship
   f. Leadership
   g. Sociability

These are not necessarily to be part of any one grade and some of them, such as those listed under social factors, are quite difficult to measure. The tools are not exceptionally valid, but there *are* tools and ways to evaluate. Again, which of these things we measure and how much weight they carry in our grade is the result of our philosophy and objectives.

There are some things which should not be part of the grade. They are: administrative problems, such as attendance, showers, and uniforms—after all, if a student misses the lesson, he should be penalized enough by missing the instruction and practice. If he did not miss anything, that's *our* fault. Showers and uniforms are important, certainly, but unless our objectives include learning to shower and learning to conform in dress, then we have no justification in grading these things. A grade should not be used as a threat; there are other ways to accomplish our ends.

We now enter a more difficult area of debate. Should we grade on effort and enthusiasm? The youngster who tries hard will do better than he would if he had not tried; his effort is reflected in his improved ability, and his enthusiasm is, in part, a result of the enthusiasm of the instructor and will also be reflected in his effort. What about improvement? After all, that is what we are seeking; that the student move to greater skill. Well, if he is classified correctly, his improvement will show up in his ability at the end of the unit. But, we say, our classes are composed of students of varying abilities. This can be solved by sub-dividing the class into, say, beginners and intermediates, teaching different skills and/or expecting different levels of performance. Our students can understand this; the gifted would be challenged and the less skilled not discouraged by having to compete for grades with those already possessing the skill they do not have.

We can, rather easily, evaluate our students at the beginning of the unit in order to place them as beginners or intermediates; then grade them according to how well they meet expectations within each group.

There will occasionally be a student who starts the unit as a beginner and, through extra effort, advances to the intermediate level rather quickly. Should we allow him to work with the intermediates even though he will now be at the bottom of that group? Obviously he would progress more if he could work with the more advanced students, and we *do* want him to progress, but it would be unfair to grade him as an intermediate. When the time comes to evaluate him, he would probably receive the highest grade as a beginner.

Motor ability is a factor which is quite measurable, but which really measures past experience and will be reflected in a student's skill. Measurement of motor ability is helpful in identifying and classifying students; and this brings up the exceptional student who is handicapped. There might be only one or two in a class, and unless the program includes a class in modified activity, we must consider that our objectives for these students are different and that our grade should be based on their ability to accomplish *those* objectives, not the objectives which have been set for the majority.

There are many grading tools which we can and should use, but probably those which will be used most will be those which the instructor devises himself. He should keep in mind that any one skill test can only measure a part of the total skill, and weigh it accordingly. Actually, well-considered subjective ratings of skill and playing ability may be the most effective and valid measures which we can use.

Subjective Evaluation

We make subjective evaluations every day, and when we are uncertain of our own ability to judge we can call upon the expert. The critic writes his column, the conductor gives a commentary, the experienced sportscaster makes his judgments, and in a learning situation, the teacher gives a grade. The teacher is an expert observer, he has the experience and background to evaluate performance. A teacher evaluates performance according to his expectations of the performer, expectations based on the learning level of the student where a performance considered good for a beginner would be only fair or poor for the advanced student.

A teacher of physical education should be an expert in basic movement skills applicable to all activities and it certainly would help if he has achieved some degree of excellence in at least *one* activity, but it must also be realized that he is usually *not* teaching the highly skilled performers. Most of his students are at beginning levels and his evaluations need not require critique of the fine points of advanced skill. In fact it is a criticism of some highly skilled teachers that their expectations of beginners are too high. This is certainly a point for argument but a teacher with some background and experience may qualify himself as an expert observer of his students.

When we were designing skill tests we used the rating of expert judges as our criterion in validating the tests; it would seem therefore that the judgment of experts is better than any skill test. Of course we used more than one expert to offset differences in emphasis, for three people evaluating a golf swing will rate the swing according to the factors which each considers most important. One may be most concerned with power and a solid contact with the ball, another may believe that a smooth, coordinated full swing is most important, while the third may not feel it necessary to have a *full* swing if stance and relative body position are maintained. These three judges might therefore assign slightly different ratings to a golfer and, for the sake of validating a test to be used by different teachers, it is necessary to use a combination of several judgments. This of course makes the skill test less than ideal for any one teacher with his particular teaching emphasis. If a teacher emphasizes a certain form or technique, and most teachers do so, then logically the students should be graded according to how well they perform under his instruction, and he then is the most expert judge of that. This is particularly true of beginning students; when students have had previous instruction from another instructor with another emphasis then there is something to be said for combined judgments and, perhaps, increased use of standardized skill tests. Of course the instructor of more advanced students presumably has had a wide variety of experience, is more aware of differing points of view regarding emphasis, and will be more cosmopolitan in his evaluations.

Methods of Assigning Grades

After giving and scoring a test the instructor is usually faced with the necessity of assigning letter grades to the scores. This is most frequently the case with written tests and skill tests. There are several systems which might be used; and which system you choose might well depend on the number and distribution of scores. If N is sufficiently large, and if the test is well constructed you should obtain a fairly normal distribution of scores with the mean close to the midpoint; and you may use any of the following systems to determine your letter grades.

TABLE 7.1 °

METHODS OF ASSIGNING GRADES

Grade	Percentage	Score	Standard Deviation
A	10	90-100	+1.5 SD and above
B	20	80-90	+0.5 SD¯ + 1.5 SD
C	40	60-80	-0.5 SD¯ + 0.5 SD
D	20	50-60	-1.5 SD¯ - 0.5 SD
F	10	Below 50	Below -1.5 SD

1. The percentage method provides a fairly normal distribution of grades and is easily applied; for example, if we have sixty students and believe them to be normally distributed in ability and accomplishment we would give 6 A's, 12 B's, 24 C's, 12 D's, and 6 F's.

2. If the score method is used A's would be assigned to scores of 90 or above, B's, to 80-90, etc. Should the test not be based on a 100 point scale the same ratios may be found by taking 10 percent of the possible score for A's, B's, and D's, and 20 percent for C's. For example if the test is based on 80 points, 10 percent would be 8 and we would have the following range:

   A = 72-80   C = 48-64   F = Below 40

   B = 64-72   D = 40-48

3. The standard deviation method assigns grades according to the number of standard deviations above or below the mean. For example, with a mean of 60 and an SD of 10 we would have the following range of grades:

   A = 75 and above (60 + 15)

   B = 65-75 (60 + 5 to 15)

C = 55-65 (60 ± 5)

D = 45-55 (60-5 to -15)

F Below 45 (60-15)

This will provide approximately 7 percent A's, 24 percent B's, 38 percent C's, 24 percent D's, and 7 percent F's, which you will note approximates the percentages of the percentage method.

PROBLEM 14

Find the final grade for the following:

	Grade	Percentage	Score
Skills			
Game Play	C	50	
Knowledge	C-	25	
Average Score	B+	25	
Grade			
Skills	B	50	
Game Play	B-	40	
Knowledge	F	10	
Average Score			
Grade			
Skills	B	50	
Game Play	B-	30	
Knowledge	F	20	
Average Score			
Grade			

4. Combinations. You may make a tally sheet of scores and apply your chosen method or use a combination of methods. As you look at the tally sheet you will probably find breaks in the continuity and should they fall close to your planned division lines it is possible to make slight adjustments in order to have definite breaks between grades. You may have a score distribution in mind but make adjustments according to the percentage method or vice versa.

The Twelve-Point Grading Scale

When we were discussing rating scales we found that it is helpful to have more than five possible ratings; this is also true when assigning grades. Although we probably will have to assign one of five letter grades in our final grade, it is helpful to use an expanded scale for the several evaluations in the course of the unit. The Twelve-Point Scale is particularly adaptable as an expansion of the traditional A, B, C, D, and F grades. It is also a useful system for rating scales. Since we think in terms of letter grades we may rate according

EXAMPLE 57

THE TWELVE POINT GRADING SCALE

Grade	Weight
A+	12
A	11
A-	10
B+	9
B	8
B-	7
C+	6
C	5
C-	4
D+	3
D	2
D-	1

to letters, or assign the numbers directly, but in either case there is a number value for each rating. It will be easier to make your cutting points when you can give plus and minus grades, for the point difference between say a B+ and an A- is not as great as that between a B and an A. This is also helpful when the distribution does not provide natural breaks, or if the scores do not assume a normal distribution.

If the distribution is not normal the standard deviation method should not be used since it is premised on a normal curve expectation, and the score method would have to be adjusted to the range of scores.

Grading Systems

How much weight we assign to the various aspects of our unit is determined by the amount of emphasis and time spent on any one factor. This of course is the result of our philosophy and possibly other circumstances such as an excessive amount of rain which necessitates spending more time on knowledges and understandings than we would under normal weather conditions.

Weights may be assigned in a numerical ratio or by percentage.

EXAMPLE 58

Factors to be Graded	Weights	Percentage
Sports Skill	3	50
Fitness	2	20
Knowledge	2	20
Concomitants	1	10

EXAMPLE 59

Factors to be Graded	Weights	Percentage
Sports Skill	2	40
Game Performance	2	40
Knowledge	1	20

There might be several skill grades to which weights could be assigned directly or they might be averaged for an average skill grade.

EXAMPLE 60
VOLLEYBALL
Using Twelve Point Scale

	Serve	Spike	Dig	Set	Skill Test	Average Skill Grade
Skill Grades	C	D+	C+	B	C-	C-
Point Score	5	3	6	8	4	26/5 = 5.2

It's possible that we would weight these items differently by counting the grades on, for example, the set and dig three times, the serve and spike two times, and the skill tests one time. In our example we would now have the following scores:

EXAMPLE 61

	Serve	Spike	Dig	Set	Skill Tests	Average Skill Grade
Skill Grades	C	D+	C+	B	C-	
Point Score	5	3	6	8	4	
Weight	2	2	3	3	1	
Weighted Score	10	6	18	24	4 =	62/11 = 5.6

Note that in order to arrive at a score on the Twelve-Point Scale we must divide by the total number of scores, in this example, eleven. Once a score has passed the top of a number, 5.5 in this case, it becomes the next higher score.

It is possible to weight grades on the various subjective ratings by having different expectations for difficult skills. For example if we feel the spike to be the most difficult skill for beginners we may not expect the same quality of performance on the spike as we expect on the other skills; in which case assigning a higher grade automatically weights the skill and all ratings may be counted equally when determining the average skill grade.

This system may also be applied to the final grade. The following are examples of possible weightings using percentages to weight the scores.

EXAMPLE 62

	Grade	Score	Percentage	Points
Skill Grades	B	8	50	400
Game Play	C+	6	30	180
Knowledges	D	2	20	40
Average Score				6.20
Grade				C+

	Grade	Score	Percentage	Points
Skill Grades	B	8	50	400
Game Play	C+	6	40	240
Knowledges	D	2	10	20
Average Score				6.60
Grade				B-

We have now reached the point where we must assign a single letter grade, and there will be some students about whom we will have to make the kind of decision which we have postponed through the use of the Twelve-Point Scale. What of the student whose final score is 6.5? Should he receive a C or a B? It's on decisions such as this that we might weigh some of the intangibles. We should consider whether or not we tend to be lenient in assigning scores and be consistent in either giving or withholding the benefit of the doubt to all students so affected.

chapter

8

Conclusion

Man thinks by manipulating symbols. The mathematician, using such symbols as ÷ and π, may think through an entire function without using a word. The symbols with which an artist thinks are even less transferable to words. Colors, shapes, light, and relationships are things which even these words fail to describe. A painting is as much an expression of thought as is an essay; and so it is for the musician composing a melody with tone and meter expressed in relationships which are auditory, and perhaps later transferred to paper through other symbols designed to represent his thought and reproduce it when followed.

Movement is perhaps the most fundamental symbolic expression, perhaps the oldest means of communication. Immense amounts of communication are achieved through gesture and posture; we need only watch an audience laughing, weeping, holding its breath in suspense while the pantomimist communicates his thoughts through movement and facial expression. Pantomime is considered to be the ultimate skill in the theatre.

When we try to execute a movement, we are trying to express a thought through movement. We think about movement with symbols which are, in part, kinesthetic. We also think in terms of form, as does the artist; we think of movement through sound (as the sound of ball and racquet meeting), and as rhythm, as does the musician. We too think in terms of angles and relationships as does the mathematician; we think of the things represented by the words force, and speed, coordination, and direction; and we think with the symbols representing the tension in our muscles, kinesthetic. All of these symbolic forms exist and are forms of communication, for the diver communicates with the spectator who understands the dive through vision, sound, verbal description, and kinesthesia; he too feels the dive in his muscles. Communication involves all of the senses, of which one is kinesthesis.

Why discuss symbolic thought in a text on measurement and evaluation? In our culture verbal communication is considered essential. Of all the skills of communication, that which is required for successful participation in the community is the ability to speak and write the language. Of course, some persons are more fluent than others, but it is certain that success is rare for the person unskilled in verbal communication, and our educational system is based on the ability to handle verbal skills. Persons skilled in other forms of communication, the performing arts, are rare. Since this is the case, it is expected that performance be translatable into words; we are expected to "describe" the picture and "discuss" the performance. "What is the artist trying to say?" "What is the moral of the play?" "What is the significance of the music?" "Write a critique" is a popular assignment in our educational system. "Evaluate." And so we try to assign words to non-verbal performances—excellent, exciting, sloppy, fair, poor. How does one evaluate a wave? It's very easy to do, for when we see it, or dive into it, we know what it is—we have made our evaluation. Now put the wave into words. That is almost impossible to do adequately, but to "evaluate the wave" *is* possible. Granted, our evaluation will be based on our expectations and experiences. A surfer can make a judgment, and the more experienced he is, the better will be his judgment; he could, if he wanted to, assign a rating to each wave—perfect, good, fair, poor. If he is a beginner on the surfboard the same waves might be rated—"yipes!", "live a little," "just my speed," and "wait for another one."

These are examples of subjective evaluation. It might also be possible to measure the wave using instruments available to oceanographers and determine its size, rate of movement, the point at which it breaks, and the temperature of the water. Such measurements represent objective evaluation. The wave may be described both subjectively and objectively and each description adds to our understanding of it, an understanding which is deeper because we have used both. In a like manner, and for the same purpose, the teacher uses both subjective and objective evaluation.

Philosophy and Evaluation

The student now has the tools at hand for constructing a program of measurement and evaluation consonant with his philosophy of evaluation, and of course his philosophy of physical education.

Most writers of texts on measurement tend toward the philosophy of realism and espouse the idea that everything is measureable in quantitative amounts, and that a grade should be founded on numerical scores arrived at through objective measurement. Such a philosophy discourages one from making subjective evaluations. The idealist, on the other hand, feels that the teacher is the best judge of ability and tends to scoff at such instruments as skill tests as being artificial and measuring parts rather than the whole performance. The pragmatist asks "does it work?" and uses whichever methods appear most useful; he would tend, however, to involve the students in the evaluative process, which neither of the others would be as likely to do. You must find your own philosophy of evaluation, probably some combination of these; all you really need is to be able to justify your methods according to a well-thought-out philosophy, and perhaps, in trying to be all things to all people use some of each in formulating your evaluative methods. Certainly your emphasis will reflect your own beliefs.

It would be pertinent to reiterate here the purposes of evaluation, for the professional student tends to become absorbed with grading and may forget that grading becomes a relatively simple task if the evaluation process has resulted in a sound program in which the students are classified properly, and in which progress is evident. These purposes—classification, determination of student status, the measurement of progress, grading, and the evaluation of program and methods—should be kept in mind when planning the physical education program. Time for measurement should be included when planning the program, and methods of evaluation should be noted. The instructor should also plan to evaluate his program and methods at appropriate intervals. Good teaching involves constant evaluation, for as we accept the good and eliminate the poor we become better teachers, and why else have we chosen this profession than that we felt we could do it well?

We should not look upon teaching as a job but rather as our life's work, the medium through which we find much of our self-realization, the good feeling that comes from doing something well. If we are good at teaching, our students benefit; if we are poor teachers no one benefits and there is no joy of accomplishment. Physical educators are fortunate to work in a field which abounds with happy things, with young people doing things which are fun to do.

The reader is finally again cautioned not to become so involved in measurement that it becomes the end rather than the means toward the accomplishment of his objectives, but by all means he should use evaluation toward the furtherance of those objectives, and toward becoming a better teacher.

Bibliograpy

GENERAL

1. Barrow, Harold M. and Rosemary McGee. *A Practical Approach to Measurement in Physical Education,* Philadelphia: Lea & Febiger, 1964.

2. Garrett, Henry E. *Statistics in Psychology and Education,* Fourth Edition, New York: Longmans, Green and Co., 1957.

3. Flanagan, John E. "General Considerations in the Solution of Test Items and a Short Method of Estimating the Product-Moment Coefficient from Data at the Tails of the Distribution," *Journal of Educational Psychology,* 1939.

4. Logsdon, Bette Jean. "A Comparison of Two Methods of Developing Physical Fitness in Fourth and Fifth Grade Girls," Unpublished dissertation, The Ohio State University, Columbus, Ohio, 1962.

5. Mathews, Donald K. *Measurement in Physical Education,* Third Edition, Philadelphia: W.B. Saunders Co., 1968.

6. Perry, Claudia K. "The Relationship Between the Presence of Lordosis and Motor Ability in College Women," Unpublished Thesis, Lamar State College of Technology, 1968.

7. Scott, M. Gladys, and Esther French. *Measurement and Evaluation in Physical Education,* Dubuque, Iowa: Wm. C. Brown Company Publishers, 1959.

TESTS
STRENGTH, ENDURANCE, FITNESS

8. AAHPER. *Youth Fitness Test Manual,* Washington, D.C.: AAHPER, 1965 (Revised).

9. Bookwalter, K.W. "Test Manual for Indiana Motor Fitness Indices for High School and College Men," *Research Quarterly*, December 1943.

10. Brouha, Lucien and J. Roswell Gallagher. "A Functional Fitness Test for High School Girls," *Journal of Health, Physical Education and Recreation*, December 1943.

11. Clarke, Harrison H. *Application of Measurement to Health and Physical Education*, Second Edition, New York: Prentice-Hall Inc., 1953.

12. Karpovich, Peter V. *Physiology of Muscular Activity*, Sixth Edition, Philadelphia: W.B. Saunders Co., 1969.

13. Kraus, Hans and Ruth P. Hirschland. "Minimum Muscular Fitness Tests in School Children," *Research Quarterly*, 25, 1954, 178-188.

14. Mathews, Donald K. *Measurement in Physical Education*, Third Edition, Philadelphia: W.B. Saunders Co., 1968.

15. State of New York. *The New York State Physical Fitness Test: A Manual for Teachers of Physical Education*, Albany, N.Y.: Division of Health, Physical Education, and Recreation, New York State Education Department, 1968.

16. Skubic, Vera and Jean Hodgkins. "A Cardiovascular Efficiency Test for Girls and Women," *Research Quarterly*, May 1963.

TESTS
MOTOR ABILITY

17. Barrow, Harold M. *Motor Ability Testing for College Men*, Minneapolis: Burgess Publishing Co., 1957.

18. ———. "Test of Motor Ability for College Men," *Research Quarterly*, 25, October 1954, 253-260.

19. Scott, M. Gladys and Esther French. *Measurement and Evaluation in Physical Education*, Dubuque, Iowa: Wm. C. Brown Co., 1959.

POSTURE

20. Kendall, Henry O., Florence P. Kendall, and Dorothy A. Boynton. *Posture and Pain*, Baltimore: The Williams and Wilkins Co., 1952.

21. State of New York. *The New York State Physical Fitness Test: A Manual for Teachers of Physical Education,* Albany, N.Y.: Division of Health, Physical Education, and Recreation, New York State Education Department, 1968.

22. Wheeler, Ruth H., and Agnes M. Hooley. *Physical Education for the Handicapped,* Philadelphia: Lea & Febiger Co., 1969.

THE CONCOMITANTS

23. Adams, R.S. "Two Scales for Measuring Attitude Toward Physical Education," *Research Quarterly,* 34, March 1963, 91-94.

24. Barrow, Harold M., and Rosemary McGee. *A Practical Approach to Measurement in Physical Education,* Philadelphia: Lea & Febiger, 1964.

25. Blanchard, B.E. Jr. "A Behavior Frequency Rating Scale for the Measurement of Character and Personality in Physical Education Classroom Situations," *Research Quarterly,* 7, May 1936, 56-66.

26. Cowell, Charles C. "Our Function is Still Education!" *The Physical Educator,* 14, March 1957, 6-7.

27. ———. "Validating an Index of Social Adjustment for High School Use," *Research Quarterly,* 29, March 1958, 7-18.

28. Haskins, Mary Jane. "Problem-Solving Test of Sportsmanship," *Research Quarterly,* 31, December 1960, 601-606.

29. Jennings, Helen. *Sociometry in Group Relations,* Washington: American Council on Education, 1948.

30. Wear, Carlos L. "The Evaluation of Attitude Toward Physical Education as an Activity Course, *Research Quarterly,* 22, March 1951, 114-126.

SPORTS SKILLS

Archery

31. AAHPER. *Archery Skills Test Manual.* Washington, D.C.: American Association for Health, Physical Education, and Recreation, 1967.

32. Hyde, Edith I. "An Achievement Scale in Archery," *Research Quarterly,* May 1937. Norms for college women using the Columbia Round.

33. Zabik, Roger M., and Andrew S. Jackson. "Reliability of Archery Achievement," *Research Quarterly,* March 1969. Analysis of Modified Chicago Round and Modified Flint Round suggests use of both measures.

Badminton

34. Lockhart, Aileene and Francis A. McPherson. "The Development of a Test of Badminton Playing Ability," *Research Quarterly,* December 1949.

    Wall Volley test. Validity .60–.71, Reliability .90.

35. Miller, Frances A. "A Badminton Wall Volley Test," *Research Quarterly,* May 1951.

    Wall Volley test. Validity .83, Reliability .94.

36. Scott, M. Gladys, Aileen Carpenter, Esther French, and Louise Kuhl. "Achievement Examinations in Badminton," *Research Quarterly,* May 1941.

    Written and skill tests with suggested grading plans and norms.

    Validities: Multiple correlations serve test and clear test .56–.85. Written test, use of item analysis provided validity. Reliabilities of skill tests .77–.98.

37. Scott, M. Gladys, and Esther French. *Measurement and Evaluation in Physical Education:* Dubuque, Iowa: Wm. C. Brown Co., 1959.

    Presentation of several skill tests and test batteries with validities.

Basketball

38. AAHPER. *Basketball Skills Test Manual for Boys,* Washington, D.C.: American Association for Health, Physical Education, and Recreation, 1966.

39. ———. *Basketball Skills Test Manual for Girls,* Washington, D.C.: American Association for Health, Physical Education, and Recreation, 1966.

40. Johnson, L.W. "Objective Tests in Basketball for High School Boys," Unpublished Master's Thesis, State University of Iowa, in Mathews, Donald K., *Measurement in Physical Education,* Third Edition, Philadelphia: W.B. Saunders Co., 1968.

    Skill Test battery. Validity .88, Reliability .89.

41. Lehsten, Carlson. "A Measure of Basketball Skills in High School Boys," *The Physical Educator,* December 1948.

    Skill Test battery. Validity .80.

42. Miller, Wilma K. "Achievement Levels in Basketball Skills for Women Physical Education Majors," *Research Quarterly,* December 1954.

    Norms established for selected basketball skills.

43. Stroup, Francis. "Game Results as a Criterion for Validating Basketball Skill Test," *Research Quarterly,* October 1955.

    Three item test battery proved effective as a predictor of game results. Team averages on battery were used. Possible use in team equalization.

Bowling

44. Martin, Joan and Jack Keogh. "Bowling Norms for College Students in Elective Physical Education Classes," *Research Quarterly,* October 1964.

    Norms established for men and women classified as a non-experienced and experienced bowlers.

45. Olson, Janice K., and Marie R. Liba. "A Device for Evaluating Spot Bowling Ability," *Research Quarterly,* May 1967.

    Describes use of an observation sheet to record point of release and point of aim.

46. Phillips, Marjorie and Dean Summers. "Bowling Norms and Learning Curves for College Women," *Research Quarterly,* December 1950.

    Norms established by level of ability and progress.

Field Hockey

47. Friedel, Jean Elizabeth. "The Development of a Field Hockey Skill Test for High School Girls, Unpublished Master's Thesis, Illinois State Normal University, in Barrow, Harold M. and Rosemary McGee, *A Practical Approach to Measurement in Physical Education,* Philadelphia: Lea & Febiger Co., 1964.

    Skill test, Validity .87 with Schmithals-French test, Reliability .77 and .90.

48. Schmithals, Margaret and Esther French. "Achievement Tests in Field Hockey for College Women," *Research Quarterly,* October 1940.

    Tests and test battery, Validities .44–.60, Reliabilities .87–.92.

Football

49. AAHPER. *Football Skills Test Manual,* Washington, D.C.: American Association for Health, Physical Education, and Recreation, 1966.

50. Borleske, Stanley E. "A Study of Achievement of College Men in Touch Football," Unpublished Master's Thesis, University of California, Berkeley, in Barrow, Harold M. and Rosemary McGee, *A Practical Approach to Measurement in Physical Education,* Philadelphia: Lea & Febiger Co., 1964.

    Test battery, Validity .88.

Golf

51. Brown, Steven H. "A Test Battery for Evaluating Golf Skills," *Texas Association for Health, Physical Education, and Recreation Journal,* May 1969.

52. McKee, Mary Ellen. "A Test for the Full-Swinging Shot in Golf," *Research Quarterly,* March 1950.

    Hard ball tests of range, velocity, and angle of impact—Acceptable Validities and Reliabilities. Soft ball test of range—Acceptable Validities and Reliabilities.

Gymnastics

53. Faulkner, John and Newt Loken. "Objectivity of Judging at the National Collegiate Athletic Association Gymnastic Meet: A Ten-Year Follow-up Study," *Research Quarterly,* October 1962.

    Use of intercorrelations in selection of judges.

54. Hunsicker, Paul and Newt Loken. "The Objectivity of Judging at the National Collegiate Athletic Association Gymnastic Meet," *Research Quarterly,* December 1951.

    Intercorrelations of judges with possibilities for changes suggested.

Handball

55. Cornish, Clayton. "A Study of Measurement of Ability in Handball," *Research Quarterly,* May 1949.

    Five skill tests, combined into test batteries—Validities of .67 and .69.

56. Pennington, Gary G.. and others. "A Measure of Handball Ability," *Research Quarterly,* May 1967.

    Test battery including service placement, wall volley, back wall placement—Validity of battery .80.

Ice Hockey

57. Merrifield, H.H. and Gerald A. Walford. "Battery of Ice Hockey Skill Tests," *Research Quarterly,* March 1969.

    Four skill tests with acceptable Validities and Reliabilities.

Soccer

58. Tomlinson, Rebecca. "Soccer Skill Test," *Soccer-Speedball Guide,* 1964-1966, Division of Girls' and Women's Sports, American Association for Health, Physical Education, and Recreation.

59. Warner, Glenn F.H. "Warner Soccer Test, Newsletter of the National Soccer Coaches Association of America, December, 1950, in Barrow, Harold M. and Rosemary McGee, *A Practical Approach to Measurement in Physical Education,* Philadelphia: Lea & Febiger Co., 1964.

Softball

60. AAHPER. *Softball Skills Test Manual for Boys,* Washington, D.C.: American Association for Health, Physical Education, and Recreation, 1966.

61. ———. *Softball Skills Test Manual for Girls,* Washington, D.C.: American Association for Health, Physical Education, and Recreation, 1966.

62. Fringer, Margaret Neal. "A Battery of Softball Skill Tests for Senior High School Girls," Unpublished Master's Thesis, University of Michigan, Ann Arbor, 1961, in Barrow, Harold M. and Rosemary McGee, *A Practical Approach to Measurement in Physical Education,* Philadelphia: Lea & Febiger Co., 1969.

    3-item battery: Validity .83, Reliabilities .72–.90.

    2-item battery: Validity .80, Reliabilities .72–87.

Swimming

63. Fox, Margaret G. "Swimming Power Test," *Research Quarterly,* October 1957.

    Test of power in front crawl and side stroke. Validities—face validity, with form .69 and .83, Reliabilities .87 and .95.

64. Hewitt, Jack E. "Swimming Achievement Scales for College Men," *Research Quarterly,* December 1948.

    Eight tests, Validities .54–.90, Reliabilities .89–.95. Short 4-item battery, Validity .87.

65. Rosentswieg, Joel. "A Revision of the Power Swimming Test," *Research Quarterly,* October 1968.

> Power tests front crawl, side, elementary back, back crawl, breast strokes, Validities—face, with form .63 to .83, Reliabilities .89 to .96.

66. Wilson, Marcia Ruth. "A Relationship Between General Motor Ability and Objective Measures of Achievement at the Intermediate Level for College Women," Unpublished Master's Thesis, The Women's College of the University of North Carolina, Greensboro, 1962.

Tennis

67. Broer, Marion R., and Donna Mae Miller. "Achievement Tests for Beginning and Intermediate Tennis," *Research Quarterly,* October 1950.

> Written test—Validities .82 beginners, .92 intermediates, Skill test, forehand and backhand drives—Validities .74-.87 intermediates, .46—.66 beginners, Reliabilities .80.

68. Dyer, Joanna Thayer. "Revision of the Backboard Test of Tennis Ability," *Research Quarterly,* March 1938.

69. Hewitt, Jack E. "Revision of the Dyer Backboard Tennis Test," *Research Quarterly,* May 1965.

70. ———. "Classification Tests in Tennis," *Research Quarterly,* October 1968.

> Two quick classification tests for use when backboard is not available.

71. Kemp, Joann and Marilyn F. Vincent. "Kemp-Vincent Rally Test of Tennis Skill," *Research Quarterly,* December 1968.

> Three minute rally between students of similar ability. Validities .84 beginners, .93 intermediates, Reliabilities .86 beginners, .90 intermediates.

72. Scott, M. Gladys and Esther French. *Measurement and Evaluation in Physical Education,* Dubuque, Iowa: Wm. C. Brown Co., 1959.

> Modification of the Dyer Test, with 27.5 foot restraining line. Scoring includes number of balls used.

Volleyball

73. AAPHER. *Volleyball Skills Test Manual,* Washington, D.C.: American Association for Health, Physical Education, and Recreation, 1969.

74. Cunningham, Phyllis and Joan Garrison. "High Wall Volley Test for Women," *Research Quarterly,* October 1968.

    Wall volley test at target. Validities .62 to .72, Reliability .87, Objectivity .83–.89.

75. Mohr, Dorothy R., and Martha J. Haverstick. "Repeated Volleys Tests in Women's Volleyball," *Research Quarterly,* May 1955.

    Wall volley test using seven foot restraining line. Validity .79, Reliability .94.

Playing Ability

76. Wright, Logan and Patsy K. Wright. "An Instrument for Evaluation of Skill in Women's Physical Education Classes," *Research Quarterly,* March 1964.

Appendix

Table of Squares (1.00 to 5.49)

(For squares of numbers between 10.0 and 54.9, move decimal point 2 places to right, etc.)

(For squares of numbers between .100 and .549, move decimal point 2 places to left, etc.)

	.00	.01	.02	.03	.04	.05	.06	.07	.08	.09
1.0	1.0000	1.0201	1.0404	1.0609	1.0816	1.1025	1.1236	1.1449	1.1664	1.1881
1.1	1.2100	1.2321	1.2544	1.2769	1.2996	1.3225	1.3456	1.3689	1.3924	1.4161
1.2	1.4400	1.4641	1.4884	1.5129	1.5376	1.5625	1.5876	1.6129	1.6384	1.6641
1.3	1.6900	1.7161	1.7424	1.7689	1.7956	1.8225	1.8496	1.8769	1.9044	1.9321
1.4	1.9600	1.9881	2.0164	2.0449	2.0736	2.1025	2.1316	2.1609	2.1904	2.2201
1.5	2.2500	2.2801	2.3104	2.3409	2.3716	2.4025	2.4336	2.4649	2.4964	2.5281
1.6	2.5600	2.5921	2.6244	2.6569	2.6896	2.7225	2.7556	2.7889	2.8224	2.8561
1.7	2.8900	2.9241	2.9584	2.9929	3.0276	3.0625	3.0976	3.1329	3.1684	3.2041
1.8	3.2400	3.2761	3.3124	3.3489	3.3856	3.4225	3.4596	3.4969	3.5344	3.5721
1.9	3.6100	3.6481	3.6864	3.7249	3.7636	3.8025	3.8416	3.8809	3.9204	3.9601
2.0	4.0000	4.0401	4.0804	4.1209	4.1616	4.2025	4.2436	4.2849	4.3264	4.3681
2.1	4.4100	4.4521	4.4944	4.5369	4.5796	4.6225	4.6656	4.7089	4.7524	4.7961
2.2	4.8400	4.8841	4.9284	4.9729	5.0176	5.0625	5.1076	5.1529	5.1984	5.2441
2.3	5.2900	5.3361	5.3824	5.4289	5.4756	5.5225	5.5696	5.6169	5.6644	5.7121
2.4	5.7600	5.8081	5.8564	5.9049	5.9536	6.0025	6.0516	6.1009	6.1504	6.2001
2.5	6.2500	6.3001	6.3504	6.4009	6.4516	6.5025	6.5536	6.6049	6.6564	6.7081
2.6	6.7600	6.8121	6.8644	6.9169	6.9696	7.0225	7.0756	7.1289	7.1824	7.2361
2.7	7.2900	7.3441	7.3984	7.4529	7.5076	7.5625	7.6176	7.6729	7.7284	7.7841
2.8	7.8400	7.8961	7.9524	8.0089	8.0656	8.1225	8.1796	8.2369	8.2944	8.3521
2.9	8.4100	8.4681	8.5264	8.5849	8.6436	8.7025	8.7616	8.8209	8.8804	8.9401
3.0	9.0000	9.0601	9.1204	9.1809	9.2416	9.3025	9.3636	9.4249	9.4864	9.5481
3.1	9.6100	9.6721	9.7344	9.7969	9.8596	9.9225	9.9856	10.0489	10.1124	10.1761
3.2	10.2400	10.3041	10.3684	10.4329	10.4976	10.5625	10.6276	10.6929	10.7584	10.8241
3.3	10.8900	10.9561	11.0224	11.0889	11.1556	11.2225	11.2896	11.3569	11.4244	11.4921
3.4	11.5600	11.6281	11.6964	11.7649	11.8336	11.9025	11.9716	12.0409	12.1104	12.1801
3.5	12.2500	12.3201	12.3904	12.4609	12.5316	12.6025	12.6736	12.7449	12.8164	12.8881
3.6	12.9600	13.0321	13.1044	13.1769	13.2496	13.3225	13.3956	13.4689	13.5424	13.6161
3.7	13.6900	13.7641	13.8384	13.9129	13.9876	14.0625	14.1376	14.2129	14.2884	14.3641
3.8	14.4400	14.5161	14.5924	14.6689	14.7456	14.8225	14.8996	14.9769	15.0544	15.1321
3.9	15.2100	15.2881	15.3664	15.4449	15.5236	15.6025	15.6816	15.7609	15.8404	15.9201
4.0	16.0000	16.0801	16.1604	16.2409	16.3216	16.4025	16.4836	16.5649	16.6464	16.7281
4.1	16.8100	16.8921	16.9744	17.0569	17.1396	17.2225	17.3056	17.3889	17.4724	17.5561
4.2	17.6400	17.7241	17.8084	17.8929	17.9776	18.0625	18.1476	18.2329	18.3184	18.4041
4.3	18.4900	18.5761	18.6624	18.7489	18.8356	18.9225	19.0096	19.0969	19.1844	19.2721
4.4	19.3600	19.4481	19.5364	19.6249	19.7136	19.8025	19.8916	19.9809	20.0704	20.1601
4.5	20.2500	20.3401	20.4304	20.5209	20.6116	20.7025	20.7936	20.8849	20.9764	21.0681
4.6	21.1600	21.2521	21.3444	21.4369	21.5296	21.6225	21.7156	21.8089	21.9024	21.9961
4.7	22.0900	22.1841	22.2784	22.3729	22.4676	22.5625	22.6576	22.7529	22.8484	22.9441
4.8	23.0400	23.1361	23.2324	23.3289	23.4256	23.5225	23.6196	23.7169	23.8144	23.9121
4.9	24.0100	24.1081	24.2064	24.3049	24.4036	24.5025	24.6016	24.7009	24.8004	24.9001
5.0	25.0000	25.1001	25.2004	25.3009	25.4016	25.5025	25.6036	25.7049	25.8064	25.9081
5.1	26.0100	26.1121	26.2144	26.3169	26.4196	26.5225	26.6256	26.7289	26.8324	26.9361
5.2	27.0400	27.1441	27.2484	27.3529	27.4576	27.5625	27.6676	27.7729	27.8784	27.9841
5.3	28.0900	28.1961	28.3024	28.4089	28.5156	28.6225	28.7296	28.8369	28.9444	29.0521
5.4	29.1600	29.2681	39.3764	29.4849	29.5936	29.7025	29.8116	29.9209	30.0304	30.1401

Table of Squares (5.50 to 9.99)

(For squares of numbers between 55.0 and 99.9, move the decimal point 2 places to the right, etc.)

(For squares of numbers between .550 and .999, move the decimal point 2 places to the left, etc.)

	.00	.01	.02	.03	.04	.05	.06	.07	.08	.09
5.5	30.2500	30.3601	30.4704	30.5809	30.6916	30.8025	30.9136	31.0249	31.1364	31.2481
5.6	31.3600	31.4721	31.5844	31.6969	31.8096	31.9225	32.0356	32.1489	32.2624	32.3761
5.7	32.4900	32.6041	32.7184	32.8329	32.9476	33.0625	33.1776	33.2929	33.4084	35.5241
5.8	33.6400	33.7561	33.8724	33.9889	34.1056	34.2225	34.3396	34.4569	34.5744	34.6921
5.9	34.8100	34.9281	35.0464	35.1649	35.2836	35.4025	35.5216	35.6409	35.7604	35.8801
6.0	36.0000	26.1201	36.2404	36.3609	36.4816	36.6025	36.7236	36.8449	36.9664	37.0881
6.1	37.2100	37.3321	37.4544	37.5769	37.6996	37.8225	37.9456	38.0689	38.1924	38.3161
6.2	38.4400	38.5641	38.6884	38.8129	38.9376	39.0625	39.1876	39.3129	39.4384	39.5641
6.3	39.6900	39.8161	39.9424	40.0689	40.1956	40.3225	40.4496	40.5769	40.7044	40.8321
6.4	40.9600	41.0881	41.2164	41.3449	41.4736	41.6025	41.7316	41.8609	41.9904	42.1201
6.5	42.2400	42.3801	42.5104	42.6409	42.7716	42.9025	43.0336	43.1649	43.2964	43.4281
6.6	43.5600	43.6921	43.8244	43.9569	44.0896	44.2225	44.3556	44.4889	44.6224	44.7561
6.7	44.8900	45.0241	45.1584	45.2929	45.4276	45.5625	45.6976	45.8329	45.9684	46.1041
6.8	46.2400	46.3761	46.5124	46.6489	46.7856	46.9225	47.0596	47.1969	47.3344	47.4721
6.9	47.6100	47.7481	47.8864	48.0249	48.1636	48.3025	48.4416	48.5809	48.7204	48.8601
7.0	49.0000	49.1401	49.2804	49.4209	49.5616	49.7025	49.8436	49.9849	50.1264	50.2681
7.1	50.4100	50.5521	50.6944	50.8369	50.9796	51.1225	51.2656	51.4089	51.5524	51.6961
7.2	51.8400	51.9841	52.1284	52.2729	52.4176	52.5625	52.7076	52.8529	52.9984	53.1441
7.3	53.2900	53.4361	53.5824	53.7289	53.8756	54.0225	54.1696	54.3169	54.4644	54.6121
7.4	54.7600	54.9081	55.0564	55.2049	55.3536	55.5025	55.6516	55.8009	55.9504	56.1001
7.5	56.2500	56.4001	56.5504	56.7009	56.8516	57.0025	57.1536	57.3049	57.4564	57.6081
7.6	57.7600	57.9121	58.0644	58.2169	58.3696	58.5225	58.6756	58.8289	58.9824	59.1361
7.7	59.2900	59.4441	59.5984	59.7529	59.9076	60.0625	60.2176	60.3729	60.5284	60.6841
7.8	60.8400	60.9961	61.1524	61.3089	61.4656	61.6225	61.7796	61.9369	62.0924	62.2521
7.9	62.4100	62.5681	62.7264	62.8849	63.0436	63.2025	63.3616	63.5209	63.6804	63.8401
8.0	64.0000	64.1601	64.3204	64.4809	64.6416	64.8025	64.9636	65.1249	65.2864	65.4481
8.1	65.6100	65.7721	65.9344	66.0969	66.2596	66.4225	66.5856	66.7489	66.9124	67.0761
8.2	67.2400	67.4041	67.5684	67.7329	67.8976	68.0625	68.2276	68.3929	68.5584	68.7241
8.3	68.8900	69.0561	69.2224	69.3889	69.5556	69.7225	69.8896	70.0569	70.2244	70.3921
8.4	70.5600	70.7281	70.8964	71.0649	71.2326	71.4025·	71.5716	71.7409	71.9104	72.0801
8.5	72.2500	72.4201	72.5904	72.7609	72.9316	73.1025	73.2736	73.4449	73.6164	73.7881
8.6	73.9600	74.1321	74.3044	74.4769	74.6496	74.8225	74.9956	75.1689	75.3424	75.5161
8.7	75.6900	75.8641	76.0384	76.2129	76.3876	76.5625	76.7376	76.9129	77.0884	77.2641
8.8	77.4400	77.6161	77.7924	77.9689	78.1456	78.3225	78.4966	78.6769	78.8544	79.0321
8.9	79.2100	79.3881	79.5664	79.7449	79.9236	80.1025	80.2816	80.4609	80.6404	80.8201
9.0	81.0000	81.1801	81.3604	81.5409	81.7216	81.9025	82.0836	82.2649	82.4464	82.6281
9.1	82.8100	82.9921	83.1744	83.3569	83.5396	83.7225	83.9056	84.0889	84.2724	84.4561
9.2	84.6400	84.8241	85.0084	85.1929	85.3776	85.5625	85.7476	85.9329	86.1184	86.3041
9.3	86.4900	86.6761	86.8624	87.0489	87.2356	87.4225	87.6096	87.7969	87.9844	88.1721
9.4	88.3600	88.5481	88.7364	88.9249	89.1136	89.3025	89.4916	89.6809	89.8704	90.0601
9.5	90.2500	90.4401	90.6304	90.8209	91.0116	91.2025	91.3936	91.5849	91.7764	91.9681
9.6	92.1600	92.3521	92.5444	92.7369	92.9296	93.1225	93.3156	93.5089	93.7024	93.8961
9.7	94.0900	94.2841	94.4784	94.6729	94.8676	95.0625	95.2576	95.4529	95.6484	95.8441
9.8	96.0400	96.2361	96.4324	96.6289	96.8256	97.0225	97.2196	97.4169	97.6144	97.8121
9.9	98.0100	98.2081	98.4064	98.6049	98.8036	99.0025	99.2016	99.4009	99.6004	99.8001

Index

AAHPER, 2
  Archery Skills Tests, 78
  Basketball Skill Tests, 90
  Fitness Test, 14
  Football Skill Tests, 115
  Softball Skill Tests, 141
  Volleyball Skill Tests, 168
Action Choice Tests, 64
Adjustment—Social, 52
Administration
  of Rating Scales, 190
  of Tests, 192
Analysis
  of Test Questions, 253
  of Multiple Choice Questions, 258
Answer Sheets, 259
Archery—Skill Tests, 78
Attitude
  Toward Physical Education, 59
  Inventory of, 60

Badminton—Skill Tests, 85
Barrow, Harold M.
  Motor Ability Test, 40
  Social Evaluation Score Card, 58
Basketball—Skill Tests, 90
Behavior, 54
  Rating Scale, 56
  Social Evaluation Score Card, 58
Blanchard, B. E., Jr.
  Behavior Rating Scale, 56
Brown, H. Steven
  Golf Skill Tests, 132

Check Lists
  Construction of, 186
  Definition of, 181
  Golf Swing, 181
  Uses of, 181
Communication
  Movement as, 274

Concomitants, 52
  Attitude, 59
  Behavior, 54
  Social Adjustment, 52
  Sportsmanship, 63
Correlation, 7, 224
  Coefficient of, 8
  Negative, 8
Cowell, Charles C.
  Personal Distance Ballot, 53
Critical Ratio (t), 222

Difference
  Between Correlated Means, 229
  Between Differences, 233
  Between Means, 219
Difficulty Rating, 225
Dyer, Joanna Thayer
  Backboard Test of Tennis Ability, 165

Endurance, 13
  Athletes—non-athletes, 13
  Testing, 13
Evaluation
  Objective, 5, 275
  Objectives of, 1
  Philosophy and, 275
  Purposes of, 275
  Subjective, 5, 180, 265, 275
Experimental Design, 234
  Examples of, 237

Field Hockey—Skill Tests, 109
Football—Skill Tests, 115

Game Performance Testing, 178
Golf
  Rating Scales, 183, 184, 185
  Skill Tests, 132
  Swing Check List, 181
Grading, 4, 262
  Measurable Factors, 263

Methods of, 267
Subjective, 265
Systems, 270
Twelve-point Scale, 269
Unhappiness with, 5
Grouping, 4

Harvard Step-up Test, 13
Rapid Form, 14
Haskins, Mary Jane
Test of Sportsmanships, 64
Hull Scale, 212

Improvement, 4, 264
Index of Discrimination, 225

Jennings, Helen H.
Sociometric Tabulation Form, 55

Karpovich, Peter V., 13
Step-up Test, 13
Kinesthesis, 274

Mean, 201
Rehability of, 216
Standard Error of, 218
Measurement
Objectives of, 1
Purpose of, 3
Median, 203
Methods, 4
Mode, 203
Motivation, 3
in Experimental Design, 236
in Testing, 119
Motor Ability, 33
Tests of, 33, 40
Movement
as Communication, 273
Kinesthesis, 274
Skill, 3

New York State Education Department
Posture Test, 45
Strength Tests, 9
Normal Curve, 204
Area Under—Table of, 207

Percentiles, 214
Philosophy
and Evaluation, 3, 275
Physical Education
Objectives of, 2
Physical Fitness, 14
Tests of, 16
Posture, 45
Tests of, 45
Screening, 49

Program, 4, 275
Progress, 4, 275

Questions
Alternate Purpose, 241
Construction of Written, 241
Difficulty Levels, 251
Difficulty Rating, 225
Essay, 249
Index of Discrimination, 255
Matching, 243
Multiple Choice, 248
Short Answer and Completion, 246
Special Format, 249

Rating Scales
Administration of, 190
Construction of, 186
Definition of, 181
Forms, 189
Golf, 183, 184, 185
Skills Inventory, 186
Student Self, 186
Tennis Serve, 189
Uses of, 181
Rehability, 7, 8
Results, Knowledge of, 4

Schmthals, Margaret
Field Hockey Skill Tests, 109
Scott, M. Gladys
Test of Motor Ability, 33
Sigma Scale, 212
Skills
Inventory, 186
Tests of, 78
Soccer Skill Test, 137
Social
Adjustment, 52
Cowell Personal Distance Ballot, 53
Status, 52, 54
Sociometric Tabulation Form, 55
Softball Skills Tests, 141
Sportsmanship, 63
Action-Choice Tests, 64
Square Root, Finding the, 209
Standard Deviation, 205
Standard Scores, 211
Sigma, Hull, T, 212
Standards, Use of. 184
Statistics
Correlation, 7, 224
Critical Ratio (t), 222
Mean, 201
Median, 203
Mode, 203
Normal Curve, 204

Percentiles, 214
Purpose of, 201
Standard Deviation, 205
Standard Error of Difference Between
     Means, 219
Standard Error of Difference Between
     Correlated Means, 229
Standard Error of Difference Between
     Differences, 233
Standard Error of the Mean, 218
Standard Scores, 211
Strength, 9
Tests of, 9
Swimming Skill Tests, 160

t (See Critical Ratio)
T Scale, 212
Team Play
Rating Scale, 186
Tennis
Skill Test, 165
Rating Scale, 189
Test
Administration, 192
Analysis, 253
Construction-questions, 241
Construction-skill, 239
Construction-written, 250
Selection, 6, 192

Tests
Archery, 78
Badminton, 85
Basketball, 90
Field Hockey, 109
Football, 115
Game Performance, 177
Golf, 132
Soccer, 137
Softball, 141
Strength, 9
Swimming, 160
Tennis, 165
Volleyball, 168
Tomlinson, Rebecca
Soccer Skill Test, 137

Validity, 7, 8, 240
Volleyball Skill Tests, 168

Wear, Carlos F.
Physical Education Attitude Inventory,
     60
Wilson, Marcia Ruth
Swimming Skill Tests, 160
Wright, Logan and Patsy K.
Basketball Scale for Women, 178